ORTHOPEDIC CLINICS OF NORTH AMERICA

www.orthopedic.theclinics.com

Surgical Considerations For Osteoporosis, Osteopenia, And Vitamin D Deficiency

July 2024 • Volume 55 • Number 3

ii

ELSEVIER

1600 John F. Kennedy Boulevard • Suite 1800 • Philadelphia, Pennsylvania, 19103-2899.

http://www.orthopedic.theclinics.com

ORTHOPEDIC CLINICS OF NORTH AMERICA Volume 55, Number 3
July 2024 ISSN 0030-5898, ISBN-13: 978-0-443-13139-4

Editor: Megan Ashdown
Developmental Editor: Shivank Joshi

Orthopedic Clinics of North America (ISSN 0030-5898) is published quarterly by Elsevier Inc., 360 Park Avenue South, New York, NY 10010-1710. Months of issue are January, April, July, and October. Business and Editorial Offices: 1600 John F. Kennedy Blvd., Suite 1800, Philadelphia, PA 19103-2899. Customer Service Office: 3251 Riverport Lane, Maryland Heights, MO 63043. Periodicals postage paid at New York, NY and additional mailing offices. Subscription prices are $368.00 per year for (US individuals), $433.00 per year (Canadian individuals), $511.00 per year (international individuals), $100.00 per year (US students), $100.00 per year for (Canadian students), $220.00 per year for (international students). For institutional access pricing please contact Customer Service via the contact information below. Foreign air speed delivery is included in all *Clinics* subscription prices. All prices are subject to change without notice. **POSTMASTER:** Send change of address to *Orthopedic Clinics of North America*, **Elsevier Health Sciences Division, Subscription Customer Service, 3251 Riverport Lane, Maryland Heights, MO 63043. Customer Service (orders, claims, online, change of address): Elsevier Health Sciences Division, Subscription Customer Service, 3251 Riverport Lane, Maryland Heights, MO 63043. Tel: 1-800-654-2452 (U.S. and Canada); 314-447-8871 (outside U.S. and Canada). Fax: 314-447-8029. E-mail:** journalscustomerservice-usa@elsevier.com **(for print support);** journalsonlinesupport-usa@elsevier.com **(for online support).**

Reprints. For copies of 100 or more, of articles in this publication, please contact the Commercial Reprints Department, Elsevier Inc., 360 Park Avenue South, New York, NY 10010-1710. Tel.: 212-633-3874; Fax: 212-633-3820; E-mail: reprints@elsevier.com.

Orthopedic Clinics of North America is covered in MEDLINE/PubMed (Index Medicus), Cinahl, Excerpta Medica, and Cumulative Index to Nursing and Allied Health Literature.

EDITORIAL BOARD

FREDERICK M. AZAR, MD – EDITOR-IN-CHIEF
Professor, Department of Orthopaedic Surgery and Biomedical Engineering, University of Tennessee-Campbell Clinic; Chief-of-Staff, Campbell Clinic, Inc, Memphis, Tennessee

WILLIAM M. MIHALKO, MD, PhD
Professor & J.R. Hyde Chair of Excellence, Chair Joint Graduate Program in Biomedical Engineering, Department of Orthopaedic Surgery & Biomedical Engineering, The University of Tennessee Health Science Center (UTHSC) - Campbell Clinic, Memphis, Tennessee

CHRISTOPHER T. COSGROVE, MD
Orthopaedic Trauma Surgery, Campbell Clinic Orthopedics, Memphis, Tennessee

MICHAEL J. BEEBE, MD
Assistant Professor, Department of Orthopaedic Surgery & Biomedical Engineering, The University of Tennessee Health Science Center (UTHSC) - Campbell Clinic, Memphis, Tennessee

BENJAMIN SHEFFER, MD
Assistant Professor, The University of Tennessee Health Science Center (UTHSC), Department of Orthopaedic Surgery, Memphis, Tennessee

JAMES H. CALANDRUCCIO, MD
Assistant Professor, Department of Orthopaedic Surgery and Biomedical Engineering, University of Tennessee-Campbell Clinic; Staff Physician, Campbell Clinic, Inc, Memphis, Tennessee

CONTRIBUTORS

EDITOR

FREDERICK M. AZAR, MD
Professor, Department of Orthopaedic
Surgery and Biomedical Engineering,
University of Tennessee-Campbell Clinic;
Chief-of-Staff, Campbell Clinic, Inc, Memphis,
Tennessee, USA

AUTHORS

JARED A. BELL, MD
Hand and Wrist Section of Orthopedic Clinics
of North America, Orthopedic Hand Fellow,
Department of Orthopaedic Surgery and
Biomedical Engineering, The University of
Tennessee Health Science Center (UTHSC) -
Campbell Clinic, Germantown, Tennessee,
USA

CLAYTON C. BETTIN, MD
Instructor, Department of Orthopaedic
Surgery and Biomedical Engineering,
University of Tennessee-Campbell Clinic;
Staff Physician, Campbell Clinic, Inc, Memphis,
Tennessee, USA

AMIT BHANDUTIA, MD
Assistant Professor, Department of
Orthopaedics, Louisiana State University
Health Sciences Center, New Orleans,
Louisiana, USA

TYLER J. BROLIN, MD
Clinical Instructor, Department of
Orthopaedic Surgery, Campbell Clinic,
University of Tennessee Health Science
Center, Memphis, Tennessee, USA

JAMES H. CALANDRUCCIO, MD
Assistant Professor, Department of
Orthopaedic Surgery and Biomedical
Engineering, University of Tennessee-
Campbell Clinic; Staff Physician, Campbell
Clinic, Inc, Memphis, Tennessee, USA

ANTONIA F. CHEN, MD, MBA
Chief of Arthroplasty and Joint
Reconstruction, Department of Orthopaedic
Surgery, Brigham and Women's Hospital,
Boston, Massachusetts, USA

TORI J. COBLE, DO
Research Scholar, Department of Orthopaedic
Surgery and Biomedical Engineering, The
University of Tennessee Health Science Center
(UTHSC) -Campbell Clinic, Germantown,
Tennessee, USA

CHRISTOPHER DEANS, MD
Assistant Professor, Department of
Orthopaedic Surgery and Rehabilitation,
University of Nebraska Medical Center,
Omaha, Nebraska, USA

ALICIA DIAZ-THOMAS, MD, MPH
Associate Professor, Division of Pediatric
Endocrinology, The University of Tennessee
Health Science Center, Division of Pediatric
Endocrinology, Le Bonheur Children's
Hospital, Memphis, Tennessee, USA

KATHERINE DONG, MD
Residents, Department of Orthopaedics,
Louisiana State University Health Sciences
Center, New Orleans, Louisiana, USA

JEREMY A. DUBIN, BA
Department of Orthopaedic Surgery, The
Rubin Institute for Advanced Orthopedics,
Sinai Hospital of Baltimore, Baltimore,
Maryland, USA

JESSICA L. DUGGAN, BS
Medical Student, Department of Orthopaedic
Surgery, Harvard Medical School, Boston,
Massachusetts, USA

WOLFGANG FITZ, MD
Department of Orthopaedic Surgery, Brigham
and Women's Hospital, Boston,
Massachusetts, USA

KEVIN L. GARVIN, MD
Professor and Chair, Department of
Orthopaedic Surgery and Rehabilitation,
University of Nebraska Medical Center,
Omaha, Nebraska, USA

DANIEL GELVEZ, MD
Residents, Department of Orthopaedics,
Louisiana State University Health Sciences
Center, New Orleans, Louisiana, USA

BENJAMIN J. GREAR, MD
Instructor, Department of Orthopaedic
Surgery and Biomedical Engineering,
University of Tennessee-Campbell Clinic;
Staff Physician, Campbell Clinic, Inc, Memphis,
Tennessee, USA

PAUL T. GREENFIELD, MD
Orthopedic Resident, Department of
Orthopaedic Surgery and Biomedical
Engineering, The University of Tennessee
Health Science Center (UTHSC) -Campbell
Clinic, Germantown, Tennessee,
USA

DANIEL HAMEED, MD
Department of Orthopaedic Surgery, Rubin
Institute for Advanced Orthopedics, Sinai
Hospital of Baltimore, Baltimore, Maryland,
USA

KEVIN A. HAO, BS
Medical Student, Department of
Orthopaedics and Rehabilitation, College of
Medicine, University of Florida, Gainesville,
Florida, USA

KEEGAN M. HONES, MD, MS
Resident, Department of Orthopaedics and
Sports Medicine, University of Florida,
Gainesville, Florida, USA

RICHARD IORIO, MD
Vice Chairman, Clinical Effectiveness Richard
D. Scott, MD, Distinguished Chair,
Department of Orthopaedic Surgery, Brigham
and Women's Hospital, Boston,
Massachusetts, USA

BEAU J. KILDOW, MD
Assistant Professor, Department of
Orthopaedic Surgery and Rehabilitation,
University of Nebraska Medical Center,
Omaha, Nebraska, USA

JOSEPH J. KING, MD
Associate Professor, Department of
Orthopaedics and Sports Medicine, University
of Florida, Gainesville, Florida, USA

JEFFREY K. LANGE, MD
Associate Orthopaedic Surgeon, Department
of Orthopaedic Surgery, Brigham and
Women's Hospital, Boston, Massachusetts,
USA

JAMES T. LAYSON, DO
Department of Orthopaedic Surgery, Lenox
Hill Hospital, New York, New York, USA

JAMES D. MICHELSON, MD
Professor, Orthopaedic Surgery, Department
of Orthopaedics and Rehabilitation, Larner
College of Medicine, University of Vermont,
Burlington, Vermont, USA

MICHAEL MONT, MD
Orthopaedic Surgeon, Department of
Orthopaedic Surgery, Rubin Institute for
Advanced Orthopedics, Sinai Hospital of
Baltimore, Baltimore, Maryland, USA

MALLORY C. MOORE, BS
Department of Orthopaedic Surgery, Rubin
Institute for Advanced Orthopedics, Sinai
Hospital of Baltimore, Baltimore, Maryland,
USA

GARNETT A. MURPHY, MD
Professor, Department of Orthopaedic
Surgery and Biomedical Engineering, The
University of Tennessee Health Science Center
(UTHSC) -Campbell Clinic, Memphis,
Tennessee, USA

ADAM OLSEN, MD
Department of Orthopaedic Surgery, Brigham
and Women's Hospital, Boston,
Massachusetts, USA

NAVEEN PATTISAPU, MD
Department of Orthopedic Surgery, Beth
Israel Lahey Hospital, Burlington,
Massachusetts, USA

NATHAN REDLICH, MD
Residents, Department of Orthopaedics,
Louisiana State University Health Sciences
Center, New Orleans, Louisiana, USA

DAVID R. RICHARDSON, MD
Professor, Department of Orthopaedic
Surgery and Biomedical Engineering, The
University of Tennessee Health Science Center
(UTHSC) -Campbell Clinic, Memphis,
Tennessee, USA

KEVIN T. ROOT, BS
College of Medicine, University of Florida,
Gainesville, Florida, USA

JORDAN D. ROSS, MD
Adult/Pediatric Endocrinology Fellow, The
University of Tennessee Health Science
Center, Memphis, Tennessee, USA

BRADLEY S. SCHOCH, MD
Associate Professor, Department of
Orthopedic Surgery, Mayo Clinic, Jacksonville,
Florida, USA

GILES R. SCUDERI, MD
Department of Orthopaedic Surgery, Lenox
Hill Hospital, New York, New York,
USA

VIVEK M. SHAH, MD
Department of Orthopaedic Surgery, Brigham
and Women's Hospital, Boston,
Massachusetts, USA

BERJE SHAMASSIAN, MD
Assistant Professor, Department of
Neurosurgery, Louisiana State University
Health Sciences Center, New Orleans,
Louisiana, USA

WILLIAM C. SKINNER, MD
Resident Physician, Department of
Orthopaedic Surgery and Biomedical
Engineering, The University of Tennessee
Health Science Center (UTHSC) -Campbell
Clinic, Memphis, Tennessee, USA

WILLIAM J. WELLER, MD
Associate Professor, Department of
Orthopaedic Surgery and Biomedical
Engineering, The University of Tennessee
Health Science Center (UTHSC) -Campbell
Clinic, Germantown, Tennessee, USA

JESTIN WILLIAMS, MD
Resident, Department of Orthopaedics,
Louisiana State University Health Sciences
Center, New Orleans, Louisiana, USA

JONATHAN O. WRIGHT, MD
Assistant professor, Department of
Orthopaedics and Sports Medicine, University
of Florida, Gainesville, Florida, USA

THOMAS W. WRIGHT, MD
Professor, Department of Orthopaedics and
Sports Medicine, University of Florida,
Gainesville, Florida, USA

JANE YEOH, MD
Orthopaedic surgeon, Department of Surgery,
Nanaimo Orthopaedics, Nanaimo, British
Columbia, Canada

BRADFORD ZITSCH, MD
Orthopaedic Surgeon, Department of
Orthopaedic Surgery and Rehabilitation,
University of Nebraska Medical Center,
Omaha, Nebraska, USA

CONTENTS

Table 2
Bivariate analysis of postoperative outcomes for total hip arthroplasty

	DEXA Cementless THA n = 17,156 (%)	DEXA Cement THA n = 6948 (%)	No DEXA Cementless THA n = 21,436 (%)	No DEXA Cement THA n = 10,061 (%)	P-value
90 d Complications					
Aseptic loosening	49 (0.29)	18 (0.26)	30 (0.14)	17 (0.17)	0.009
Blood transfusion	290 (1.69)	151 (2.17)	325 (1.52)	196 (1.95)	0.001
Cardiac arrest	15 (0.09)	a	12 (0.06)	13 (0.13)	0.164
CVA	114 (0.66)	80 (1.15)	128 (0.60)	79 (0.79)	<0.001
Dislocation	175 (1.02)	62 (0.89)	186 (0.87)	74 (0.74)	0.107
DVT	227 (1.32)	105 (1.51)	229 (1.07)	133 (1.32)	0.013
MI	95 (0.55)	54 (0.78)	92 (0.43)	68 (0.68)	0.002
PE	97 (0.57)	59 (0.85)	132 (0.62)	65 (0.65)	0.089
PJI	176 (1.03)	126 (1.81)	226 (1.05)	125 (1.24)	<0.001
PNA	450 (2.62)	242 (3.48)	485 (2.26)	327 (3.25)	<0.001
PPFx	130 (0.76)	50 (0.72)	132 (0.62)	54 (0.54)	0.119
Renal failure	212 (1.24)	107 (1.54)	173 (0.81)	149 (1.48)	<0.001
Revision	152 (0.89)	55 (0.79)	126 (0.59)	57 (0.57)	0.001
SSI	193 (1.12)	96 (1.38)	188 (0.88)	104 (1.03)	0.002
1 y Complications					
Aseptic loosening	85 (0.50)	26 (0.37)	61 (0.28)	35 (0.35)	0.009
Dislocation	293 (1.71)	123 (1.77)	331 (1.54)	122 (1.21)	0.006
Mechanical	87 (0.51)	26 (0.37)	110 (0.51)	39 (0.39)	0.244
PJI	328 (1.91)	208 (2.99)	393 (1.83)	217 (2.16)	<0.001
PPFx	234 (1.36)	91 (1.31)	241 (1.12)	103 (1.02)	0.041
Revision	280 (1.63)	89 (1.28)	239 (1.11)	103 (1.02)	<0.001
SSI	384 (2.24)	183 (2.63)	360 (1.68)	198 (1.97)	<0.001
2 y Complications					
Aseptic loosening	96 (0.56)	36 (0.52)	80 (0.37)	46 (0.46)	0.053
Dislocation	369 (2.15)	151 (2.17)	421 (1.96)	165 (1.64)	0.020
PJI	420 (2.45)	244 (3.51)	522 (2.44)	296 (2.94)	<0.001
PPFx	307 (1.79)	122 (1.76)	316 (1.47)	142 (1.41)	0.024
Revision	340 (1.98)	111 (1.60)	321 (1.50)	132 (1.31)	<0.001

Abbreviations: CVA, cerebrovascular accident; DVT, deep vein thrombosis; MI, myocardial infarction; PE, pulmonary embolism; PJI, prosthetic joint infection; PNA, pneumonia; PPFx, periprosthetic fracture; SSI, surgical site infection; THA, total hip arthroplasty.
a Censored in accordance with the database confidentiality agreement.

(CHF), cerebrovascular disease (CVD), rheumatoid arthritis (RA), liver disease, and tobacco use.

Patient Selection
The patients were then categorized by 2 methods. First patients were identified by type of femoral stem fixation, cementless or cemented. They were also differentiated by whether DEXA scan was performed preoperatively by using CPT codes 77080 and 77081. It was postulated that patients who had a preoperative DEXA scan had a higher probability of osteoporosis compared to those patients who did not have a scan. Patients were therefore differentiated into 4 different subsets: DEXA cementless, DEXA cemented, no DEXA cementless, and no DEXA cemented.

Using these patients, complication rates were tabulated via ICD and CPT codes. For this study,

Table 3
Odds ratios of complications after total hip arthroplasty

	DEXA Cement THA		No DEXA Cementless THA		No DEXA Cement THA n = 10,061 (%)	
	OR	95% CI	OR	95% CI	OR	95% CI
90 d Complications						
Aseptic loosening	0.91	0.53–1.56	0.49	0.31–0.77	0.59	0.34–1.03
Blood transfusion	1.29	1.06–1.58	0.90	0.76–1.05	1.16	0.96–1.39
Cardiac arrest	1.32	0.56–3.11	0.64	0.30–1.37	1.48	0.70–3.11
CVA	1.74	1.31–2.32	0.90	0.70–1.16	1.18	0.89–1.58
Dislocation	0.87	0.65–1.17	0.85	0.69–1.05	0.72	0.55–0.94
DVT	1.14	0.91–1.44	0.81	0.67–0.97	1.00	0.81–1.24
MI	1.41	1.01–1.97	0.77	0.58–1.03	1.22	0.89–1.67
PE	1.51	1.09–2.08	1.09	0.84–1.42	1.14	0.83–1.57
PJI	1.78	1.42–2.24	1.03	0.84–1.25	1.21	0.96–1.53
PNA	1.34	1.14–1.57	0.86	0.75–0.98	1.25	1.08–1.44
PPFx	0.95	0.68–1.32	0.81	0.64–1.03	0.71	0.51–0.97
Renal failure	1.25	0.99–1.58	0.65	0.53–0.80	1.20	0.97–1.48
Revision	0.89	0.65–1.22	0.66	0.52–0.84	0.64	0.47–0.87
SSI	1.23	0.96–1.58	0.78	0.64–0.95	0.92	0.72–1.17
1 y Complications						
Aseptic loosening	0.75	0.49–1.17	0.57	0.41–0.80	0.70	0.47–1.04
Dislocation	1.04	0.84–1.28	0.90	0.77–1.06	0.71	0.57–0.87
Mechanical	0.74	0.48–1.14	1.01	0.76–1.34	0.76	0.52–1.11
PJI	1.58	1.33–1.89	0.96	0.83–1.11	1.13	0.95–1.34
PPFx	0.96	0.75–1.22	0.82	0.69–0.99	0.75	0.59–0.94
Revision	0.78	0.62–0.99	0.68	0.57–0.81	0.62	0.50–0.78
SSI	1.18	0.99–1.41	0.75	0.65–0.86	0.88	0.74–1.04
2 y Complications						
Aseptic loosening	0.93	0.63–1.36	0.67	0.49–0.90	0.82	0.57–1.16
Dislocation	1.01	0.83–1.22	0.91	0.79–1.05	0.76	0.63–0.91
PJI	1.45	1.24–1.70	0.99	0.87–1.13	1.21	1.04–1.40
PPFx	0.98	0.79–1.21	0.82	0.70–0.96	0.79	0.64–0.96
Revision	0.80	0.65–1.00	0.75	0.64–0.88	0.66	0.54–0.81

Abbreviations: 95% CI, 95% confidence interval; CVA, cerebrovascular accident; DVT, deep vein thrombosis; MI, myocardial infarction; OR, odds ratio; PE, pulmonary embolism; PJI, prosthetic joint infection; PNA, pneumonia; PPFx, periprosthetic fracture; SSI, surgical site infection; THA, total hip arthroplasty.
    Referent group: DEXA cementless THA.

these included PPFFx (CPT 27514), aseptic loosening (CPT 27137 and 27138), and prosthetic joint infections (PJIs; ICD T84.5). These codes were collected at multiple time intervals: 90 days, 1 year, and 2 years.

Demographics

Baseline characteristics were compared among groups (**Table 1**). Overall, 88.4% of patients were female individuals, which was as anticipated for a patient population with osteoporosis. In the overall patient population, the comorbidities included 6.3% who had alcohol (ETOH) abuse, 16.4% who had CCI greater than 3, 40% who had DM, 29% who had obesity and CKD, 24.5% who had cancer, 5.8% who had metastatic cancer, 22.7% who had solid tumor without metastasis, 13% who had CHF, 37.3% who had CVD,

Table 4
Multivariate logistic regression for prosthetic joint infection

	OR[a]	95% CI	P-value
90 d PJI			
Male sex	1.04	0.94–1.15	.410
Alcohol abuse	1.73	1.57–1.91	<.001
CKD	1.62	1.52–1.72	<.001
Cancer	0.91	0.73–1.13	.418
Metastatic cancer	0.88	0.78–1.00	.049
Solid tumor without metastasis	1.32	1.07–1.66	.013
CVD	1.21	1.14–1.28	<.001
CHF	0.73	0.67–0.79	<.001
Diabetes mellitus	1.14	1.07–1.22	<.001
Severe liver disease	1.05	0.86–1.28	.611
Obesity	2.16	2.03–2.29	<.001
RA	3.33	3.13–3.55	<.001
Tobacco use	1.20	1.13–1.27	<.001
DEXA cementless THA	0.76	0.71–0.82	<.001
DEXA cement THA	1.23	1.11–1.36	<.001
1 y PJI			
Male sex	0.97	0.90–1.05	.460
Alcohol abuse	1.68	1.55–1.81	<.001
CKD	1.50	1.43–1.58	<.001
Cancer	1.57	1.37–1.79	<.001
Metastatic cancer	1.10	1.00–1.21	.054
Solid tumor without metastasis	0.64	0.56–0.74	<.001
CVD	1.00	0.95–1.05	.957
CHF	1.08	1.02–1.15	.014
Diabetes mellitus	1.13	1.08–1.19	<.001
Severe liver disease	1.29	1.11–1.49	.001
Obesity	2.02	1.92–2.12	<.001
RA	3.04	2.89–3.20	<.001
Tobacco use	1.30	1.24–1.37	<.001
DEXA cementless THA	0.96	0.90–1.02	.177
DEXA cement THA	1.38	1.28–1.50	<.001
2-y PJI			
Male sex	1.02	0.95–1.09	.668
Alcohol abuse	1.93	1.79–2.07	<.001
CKD	1.47	1.40–1.54	<.001
Cancer	1.32	1.15–1.50	<.001
Metastatic cancer	1.22	1.12–1.33	<.001
Solid tumor without metastasis	0.72	0.63–0.83	<.001
CVD	1.02	0.98–1.07	.301
CHF	1.06	1.00–1.12	.044

(continued on next page)

	OR[a]	95% CI	P-value
Diabetes mellitus	1.13	1.08–1.18	<.001
Severe liver disease	1.37	1.20–1.56	<.001
Obesity	1.94	1.85–2.03	<.001
RA	2.95	2.81–3.09	<.001
Tobacco use	1.27	1.22–1.33	<.001
DEXA cementless THA	0.96	0.91–1.02	.211
DEXA cement THA	1.20	1.11–1.29	<.001

Abbreviations: 95% CI, 95% confidence interval; CHF, congestive heart failure; CKD, chronic kidney disease; CVD, cerebrovascular disease; OR, odds ratio; PJI, prosthetic joint infection; PPFx, periprosthetic fracture; RA, rheumatoid arthritis; THA, total hip arthroplasty.
[a] Referent groups: No DEXA cementless THA; No DEXA cement THA.

10.1% who had RA, 1.2% who had severe liver disease, and 44.9% who had tobacco use.

Statistical Analyses

Continuous variables such as age were compared using Student t test. Categorical variables, including demographics, comorbidities, and complications utilized chi-squared test in bivariate analyses. Complications were compared among the 4 groups, using unadjusted odds ratios (ORs) with 95% confidence intervals (CIs). Additionally, multivariate logistic regressions were performed to analyze independent risk factors for periprosthetic fractures, aseptic loosening, and PJIs among the groups. The study was granted exemption status by the local institutional review board. All analyses were performed using R Studio (Statistics Department of the University of Auckland, New Zealand) with significance regarded as $P<.05$.

RESULTS

Overall, 55,601 patients that underwent THA were included in the study. For patients with DEXA scans, there were 17,156 patients in the DEXA cementless and 6948 patients in the DEXA cement groups, respectively. In the groups without DEXA scans, there were 21,436 patients in the cementless and 10,061 patients in the cement groups, respectively.

Bivariate analysis was then performed of 90 day, 1 year, and 2 year complication rates (Table 2). ORs were performed with DEXA cementless group as the control (Table 3). Though group baseline characteristics varied, there were higher rates of aseptic loosening and PPFFx noted in patients with DEXA scans regardless of femoral fixation.

For the rest of the analysis, multivariate regression was performed. For PJI, statistically significant risk factors included ETOH abuse, CKD, solid tumor without metastasis, CHF, DM, obesity, RA, and tobacco use across all time periods (Table 4). CVD was a risk factor only in the 90 day period, whereas cancer and severe liver disease were risk factors only at 1 year and 2 year periods. The cement DEXA group was at risk for PJI compared to the cementless group at 1 year and 2 years, but no difference in 90 day PJI.

In regards to PPFFx, ETOH abuse, CKD, CVD, CHF, RA, and tobacco use were significant risk factors (Table 5). Diabetes was statistically significant in the 90 day period, and liver disease was significant in the 1 and 2 year periods. In all time periods, patients who had DEXA scans were at an increased risk for PPFFx, regardless of cementless versus cemented fixation.

Finally, for aseptic loosening, ETOH abuse, CKD, CVD, obesity, and RA were risk factors at all time periods (Table 6). Solid tumor without metastasis was a risk factor only at the 90 day period. In the first 90 days, there was no difference in aseptic loosening for patients with osteoporosis based on cementless or cemented fixation. However, there were increased rates of aseptic loosening at 1 year and 2 year time periods for the cementless fixation group with DEXA scans.

DISCUSSION

In our study, we demonstrated that patients with osteoporosis who had comorbidities of ETOH abuse, CKD, CVD, obesity, and RA continue to be at significant risk for complications following THA. Patients who had DEXA scans were at an

Table 5
Multivariate logistic regression for periprosthetic fracture

	OR[a]	95% CI	P-value
90 d PPFx			
Male sex	1.13	0.99–1.28	.060
Alcohol abuse	2.76	2.46–3.09	<.001
CKD	1.15	1.06–1.25	.001
Cancer	0.81	0.61–1.06	.142
Metastatic cancer	0.91	0.77–1.08	.283
Solid tumor without metastasis	1.27	0.96–1.71	.102
CVD	1.53	1.42–1.65	<.001
CHF	1.27	1.15–1.40	<.001
Diabetes mellitus	0.85	0.78–0.92	<.001
Severe liver disease	0.84	0.63–1.10	.230
Obesity	0.86	0.79–0.94	.001
RA	2.26	2.07–2.46	<.001
Tobacco use	0.68	0.63–0.74	<.001
DEXA cementless THA	1.51	1.37–1.68	<.001
DEXA cement THA	1.42	1.24–1.62	<.001
1 y PPFx			
Male sex	1.07	0.96–1.18	.215
Alcohol abuse	2.41	2.19–2.64	<.001
CKD	1.16	1.09–1.24	<.001
Cancer	1.16	0.96–1.39	.123
Metastatic cancer	1.02	0.89–1.16	.766
Solid tumor without Metastasis	0.80	0.66–0.97	.023
CVD	1.35	1.27–1.43	<.001
CHF	1.19	1.10–1.29	<.001
Diabetes mellitus	0.99	0.93–1.05	.642
Severe liver disease	0.55	0.42–0.72	<.001
Obesity	1.06	0.99–1.13	.107
RA	1.82	1.70–1.96	<.001
Tobacco use	0.78	0.73–0.83	<.001
DEXA cementless THA	1.38	1.28–1.49	<.001
DEXA cement THA	1.27	1.14–1.42	<.001
2 y PPFx			
Male sex	1.03	0.94–1.13	.474
Alcohol abuse	2.17	1.99–2.37	<.001
CKD	1.29	1.22–1.37	<.001
Cancer	1.13	0.94–1.34	.177
Metastatic cancer	0.88	0.78–0.99	.035
Solid tumor without metastasis	0.92	0.77–1.11	.350
CVD	1.34	1.27–1.41	<.001
CHF	1.10	1.02–1.18	.011

(continued on next page)

	OR[a]	95% CI	P-value
Diabetes mellitus	1.04	0.98–1.10	.233
Severe liver disease	0.66	0.52–0.82	<.001
Obesity	1.07	1.01–1.14	.028
RA	1.92	1.79–2.04	<.001
Tobacco use	0.90	0.85–0.95	<.001
DEXA cementless THA	1.17	1.09–1.25	<.001
DEXA cement THA	1.18	1.06–1.30	.002

Abbreviations: 95% CI, 95% confidence interval; CHF, congestive heart failure; CKD, chronic kidney disease; CVD, cerebrovascular disease; OR, odds ratio; PJI, prosthetic joint infection; PPFx, periprosthetic fracture; RA, rheumatoid arthritis; THA, total hip arthroplasty.
[a] Referent groups: No DEXA cementless THA; No DEXA cement THA.

increased risk for PPFFx regardless of femoral fixation method, and patients who had DEXA scans with cementless fixation were at risk of aseptic loosening. In this study, patients who had DEXA scans presumably had a higher severity of osteoporosis, necessitating a further osteoporotic workup. Therefore, these patients with severe osteoporosis may have higher risks for aseptic loosening and PPFFx.

It has been clear that patients with osteoporosis are at an increased risk of periprosthetic fracture .[10,11] These patients generally have Dorr C type femoral canals, which have also demonstrated increased PPFFx risk.[20,21] However, patients undergoing treatment of osteoporosis and focus on bone health can potentially diminish risks for this population with osteoporosis.[22] Cohen and colleagues demonstrated a decreased incidence of PPFFx for patients treated for osteoporosis treated with arthroplasty following a hip fracture. In their study, the 10 year incidence was 3.88% for treated patients versus 5.92% for those who were untreated.[23]

In this study, the cemented DEXA group was at risk for 90 day PJI, but not at any other time points. Though treatment of osteoporosis can significantly reduce the revision risk and increase implant survival in the population with osteoporosis, bisphosphonate treatment could potentially increase the risk of revision due to deep infection.[24–26] This has been postulated to be due to the necessity of osteoclastic resorption to help dispose of the necrotic bone surrounding an infection.[27]

Outside of this, our study demonstrated cementless fixation in the population with DEXA scans had increased rates of aseptic loosening at 1 year and 2 year intervals. Treatment of osteoporosis may inhibit osteointegration, which is critical in patients undergoing cementless arthroplasty to mitigate the possibility of mechanical loosening.[28] It is also important to recognize that, as a whole, patients with osteoporosis have abnormal bony remodeling, potentially affecting ingrowth. Due to this, it may be wise to consider cemented femoral fixation in this population undergoing elective THA. Yang and colleagues demonstrated a lower aseptic loosening rate at 5 year follow-up in cemented THA compared to cementless THA in an osteoporotic cohort.[29] As previously discussed, these patients with severe osteoporosis may have been more likely to have had treatment, potentially leading to the increased aseptic loosening rates in the group with DEXA scans.

Our study demonstrated patients who had DEXA scans were at an increased risk of PPFFx and aseptic loosening. As to why these patients receiving DEXA scans are at-risk lends to a few possibilities. Though bone mineral density T-score less than 2.5 defines osteoporosis according to the World Health Organization, it may also be determined by the presence of a fragility fracture.[30] These patients may have had a prior fragility fracture injury, which then necessitated further osteoporotic workup to include a DEXA scan to assess their bone mineral density. These patients may also have a frail general appearance and more comorbidities (in this study, patients with DEXA scans had a higher CCI), leading to further protective diagnostics to guide treatment. And as discussed, they may have had treatment with medication, either in the past or in the perioperative period, potentially putting them at an increased risk compared to the reference group.

Table 6
Multivariate logistic regression for aseptic loosening

	OR[a]	95% CI	P-value
90 d Aseptic loosening			
Male sex	0.82	0.66–1.01	.071
Alcohol abuse	5.60	4.81–6.50	<.001
CKD	2.03	1.79–2.31	<.001
Cancer	0.96	0.59–1.47	.872
Metastatic cancer	1.04	0.82–1.29	.765
Solid tumor without metastasis	1.69	1.10–2.75	.025
CVD	2.04	1.79–2.32	<.001
CHF	1.05	0.89–1.23	.566
Diabetes mellitus	0.91	0.80–1.04	.166
Obesity	1.31	1.15–1.51	<.001
RA	1.29	1.10–1.52	.002
Tobacco use	0.83	0.73–0.95	.006
DEXA cementless THA	1.88	1.59–2.25	<.001
DEXA cement THA	1.71	1.35–2.18	<.001
1 y Aseptic loosening			
Male sex	0.83	0.69–0.99	.038
Alcohol abuse	3.39	2.95–3.89	<.001
CKD	1.47	1.32–1.63	<.001
Cancer	1.14	0.79–1.59	.470
Metastatic cancer	0.86	0.70–1.05	.149
Solid tumor without metastasis	1.31	0.93–1.90	.142
CVD	1.56	1.41–1.73	<.001
CHF	1.04	0.91–1.19	.570
Diabetes mellitus	1.05	0.94–1.17	.378
Severe liver disease	0.46	0.28–0.70	.001
Obesity	1.28	1.15–1.43	<.001
RA	1.44	1.27–1.64	<.001
Tobacco use	1.01	0.91–1.12	.907
DEXA cementless THA	1.60	1.40–1.83	<.001
DEXA cement THA	0.95	0.79–1.15	.580
2 y Aseptic loosening			
Male sex	1.04	0.89–1.21	.601
Alcohol abuse	3.43	3.01–3.90	<.001
CKD	1.38	1.25–1.53	<.001
Cancer	1.09	0.77–1.50	.591
Metastatic cancer	0.81	0.66–0.98	.035
Solid tumor without metastasis	1.29	0.93–1.83	.144
CVD	1.37	1.24–1.50	<.001
CHF	1.09	0.96–1.24	.175
Diabetes mellitus	1.03	0.94–1.14	.504

(continued on next page)

	OR[a]	95% CI	P-value
Severe liver disease	0.82	0.58–1.11	.217
Obesity	1.42	1.28–1.57	<.001
RA	1.43	1.26–1.61	<.001
Tobacco use	0.98	0.89–1.08	.696
DEXA cementless THA	1.48	1.31–1.68	<.001
DEXA cement THA	0.95	0.80–1.12	.542

Abbreviations: 95% CI, 95% confidence interval; CHF, congestive heart failure; CKD, chronic kidney disease; CVD, cerebrovascular disease; OR, odds ratio; PJI, prosthetic joint infection; PPFx, periprosthetic fracture; RA, rheumatoid arthritis; THA, total hip arthroplasty.

[a] Referent groups: No DEXA cementless THA; No DEXA cement THA.

With the potential utility of the DEXA scan in identifying patients with severe osteoporosis, it is important to consider what preventative measures could be implemented. First, it is important to recognize that there is a high prevalence of undertreatment of osteoporosis for patients receiving THA, with one study demonstrating 73% of patients who had osteoporosis were not diagnosed until their preoperative DEXA scan.[18] Bernatz and colleagues showed in their series that though 25% of patients met criteria for medication treatment, only 5% received these medications in the perioperative period.[19] We have previously discussed that bisphosphonate treatment can significantly reduce the revision risk and increase implant survival in the population with osteoporosis.[24–26] It may also be beneficial to consider cemented THA in these patients who had severe osteoporosis.

The authors acknowledge potential limitations of the study, including, the retrospective nature of the study. As with any database study, there are inherent limitations. Proper diagnostic coding and categorization of patients is critical for any accuracy of a database study, which cannot be ensured. Definitions of complications and comorbidities can vary between providers and health systems. Patients receiving treatment of osteoporosis were not tracked, but may be a future point of study. Also, all patients in the study had a baseline diagnosis of osteoporosis, and were assumed to have a higher severity of osteoporosis that potentially facilitated workup with DEXA scan. Since all patients did not have DEXA scans, it is not possible to compare the severity level directly. The strength of our studies lies in the evaluation of the use of DEXA scans in conjunction with cementless and cemented THA to aid in prognosis in patients who had osteoporosis utilizing large patient numbers in a nationally representative database.

SUMMARY

This report provides an updated analysis for patients with osteoporosis. The comorbidities of ETOH abuse, CKD, CVD, obesity, and RA continue to be significant risk factors for PPFFx and aseptic loosening in the population with osteoporosis. Patients who had DEXA scans were at an increased risk for PPFFx regardless of femoral fixation method, and patients who had DEXA scans with cementless fixation were at risk of aseptic loosening. The population with severe osteoporosis may have higher risks for aseptic loosening and PPFFx than previously recognized.

CLINICS CARE POINTS

- Osteoporotic patients continue to be an "at-risk" population- Following THA, these patients are at higher risk for complications.
- In this study, patients with DEXA scans were at higher risk for aseptic loosening and PPFFx.
- DEXA scans may have utility in determining at-risk patients with severe osteoporosis, and may be useful in determining femoral fixation during THA.

REFERENCES

1. Kurtz SM, Ong K, Lau E, et al. Projections of Primary and Revision Hip and Knee Arthroplasty in the United States from 2005 to 2030. J Bone Jt Surg Am Vol 2007;89(4):780–5.
2. Schwartz AM, Farley KX, Guild GN, et al. Projections and Epidemiology of Revision Hip and Knee Arthroplasty in the United States to 2030. J Arthroplasty 2020;35(6):S79–85.

3. Callaghan JJ, Albright JC, Goetz DD, et al. Charnley Total Hip Arthroplasty with Cement. J Bone Jt Surg Am Vol 2000;82(4):487–97.

4. Donaldson A, Thomson H, Harper NJN, et al. Bone cement implantation syndrome. Br J Addiction: Br J Anaesth 2009;102(1):12–22.

5. Diehl P, Haenle M, Bergschmidt Philipp, et al. Zementfreie Hüftendoprothetik: eine aktuelle Übersicht/Cementless total hip arthroplasty: a review. Biomed Tech 2010;55(5):251–64.

6. The AJRR Annual Report. (2022). Aaos.org. Available at: https://www.aaos.org/registries/publications/ajrr-annual-report/.

7. Stihsen C, Springer B, Nemecek E, et al. Cementless Total Hip Arthroplasty in Octogenarians. J Arthroplasty 2017;32(6):1923–9.

8. Keisu KS, Orozco F, Sharkey PF, et al. Primary Cementless Total Hip Arthroplasty in Octogenarians. J Bone Joint Surg 2023;83(3):359.

9. Springer BD, Etkin CD, Shores P, et al. Perioperative Periprosthetic Femur Fractures are Strongly Correlated With Fixation Method: an Analysis From the American Joint Replacement Registry. J Arthroplasty 2019;34(7):S352–4.

10. Binkley N, Nickel BT, Anderson PA. Periprosthetic fractures: an unrecognized osteoporosis crisis. Osteoporosis International 2023;34(6):1055–64.

11. Sidler-Maier CC, Waddell JP. Incidence and predisposing factors of periprosthetic proximal femoral fractures: a literature review. Int Orthop 2015; 39(9):1673–82.

12. Fiedler B, Patel V, Lygrisse KA, et al. The effect of reduced bone mineral density on elective total hip arthroplasty outcomes. Arch Orthop Trauma Surg 2023;143(9):5993–9.

13. Shen TS, Gu A, Bovonratwet Patawut, et al. Etiology and Complications of Early Aseptic Revision Total Hip Arthroplasty Within 90 Days. J Arthroplasty 2021;36(5):1734–9.

14. Stuart Melvin J, Karthikeyan T, Cope R, et al. Early Failures in Total Hip Arthroplasty — A Changing Paradigm. J Arthroplasty 2014;29(6):1285–8.

15. Wyles CC, Maradit-Kremers H, Fruth KM, et al. Frank Stinchfield Award: Creation of a Patient-Specific Total Hip Arthroplasty Periprosthetic Fracture Risk Calculator. J Arthroplasty 2023;38(7):S2–10.

16. Islam R, Lanting BA, Somerville L, et al. Evaluating the Functional and Psychological Outcomes Following Periprosthetic Femoral Fracture After Total Hip Arthroplasty. Arthroplasty Today 2022;18:57–62.

17. Turnbull G, Scott CEH, MacDonald DJ, et al. Return to activity following revision total hip arthroplasty. Arch Orthop Trauma Surg 2018;139(3):411–21.

18. Delsmann MM, Strahl A, Mühlenfeld M, et al. High prevalence and undertreatment of osteoporosis in elderly patients undergoing total hip arthroplasty. Osteoporosis International 2021;32(8):1661–8.

19. Bernatz JT, Brooks AE, Squire MW, et al. Osteoporosis Is Common and Undertreated Prior to Total Joint Arthroplasty. J Arthroplasty 2019;34(7):1347–53.

20. Nash W, Harris A. The Dorr Type and Cortical Thickness Index of the Proximal Femur for Predicting Peri-Operative Complications during Hemiarthroplasty. J Orthop Surg 2014;22(1):92–5.

21. Gromov K, Buhl Bersang A, Nielsen CS, et al. Risk factors for post-operative periprosthetic fractures following primary total hip arthroplasty with a proximally coated double-tapered cementless femoral component. The Bone & Joint Journal 2017;99-B(4):451–7.

22. Karachalios T, Koutalos A, Komnos G. Total hip arthroplasty in patients with osteoporosis. Hip Int 2019;30(4):370–9.

23. Cohen JS, Agarwal AR, Kinnard MJ, et al. The Association of Postoperative Osteoporosis Therapy With Periprosthetic Fracture Risk in Patients Undergoing Arthroplasty for Femoral Neck Fractures. J Arthroplasty 2023;38(4):726–31.

24. Prieto-Alhambra D, Javaid MK, Judge A, et al. Association between bisphosphonate use and implant survival after primary total arthroplasty of the knee or hip: population based retrospective cohort study. BMJ 2011;343(dec06 1):d7222.

25. Thillemann TM, Pedersen AB, Mehnert F, et al. Postoperative use of bisphosphonates and risk of revision after primary total hip arthroplasty: A nationwide population-based study. Bone 2010; 46(4):946–51.

26. Khatod M, Inacio MCS, Dell R, et al. Association of Bisphosphonate Use and Risk of Revision After THA: Outcomes From a US Total Joint Replacement Registry. Clin Orthop Relat Res 2015;473(11): 3412–20.

27. Gromov K., Huang W., Li D., et al., 2008 Osteoclastic bone resorption in chronic osteomyelitis. In: The Danish Orthopaedic Society's Annual Meeting. Denmark in 2008. (ed.).

28. Russell L. Osteoporosis and Orthopedic Surgery: Effect of Bone Health on Total Joint Arthroplasty Outcome. Curr Rheumatol Rep 2013;15(11). https://doi.org/10.1007/s11926-013-0371-x.

29. Yang C, Han X, Wang J, et al. Cemented versus uncemented femoral component total hip arthroplasty in elderly patients with primary osteoporosis: retrospective analysis with 5-year follow-up. J Int Med Res 2019;47(4):1610–9.

30. Sözen T, Özışık L, Başaran NÇ. An overview and management of osteoporosis. European Journal of Rheumatology 2017;4(1):46–56.

Postoperative Vitamin D Surveillance and Supplementation in Revision Total Knee Arthroplasty Patients
A Retrospective Cohort Analysis

Jessica L. Duggan, BS[a],*, Wolfgang Fitz, MD[b],
Jeffrey K. Lange, MD[b], Vivek M. Shah, MD[b],
Adam Olsen, MD[b], Richard Iorio, MD[b],
Antonia F. Chen, MD, MBA[b]

KEYWORDS

- Revision arthroplasty • Revision total knee arthroplasty • Vitamin D • Vitamin D deficiency
- Complications • Postoperative care

KEY POINTS

- Unexpectedly, patients who were prescribed vitamin D supplementation showed significantly lower vitamin D levels postoperatively at 3 months and 1 year when compared to their baseline levels.
- In comparing dose regimens, the high-dose group showed lower vitamin D levels at 2 years compared to the no supplementation group.
- Around 57% of patients had vitamin D deficiency at any time point. Patients with vitamin D deficiency were significantly younger in age when compared to vitamin D sufficient patients.
- In total, 54% of vitamin D deficient patients achieved repletion, and the average time to repletion was 12.00 ± 7.75 months.
- Female sex was associated with low or medium dose regimens, while male sex was associated with no supplementation (*P* = .024).

INTRODUCTION

Over the last several decades, evidence has shown that vitamin D (also known as calcitriol, or 1,25-OH vitamin D) plays an important role in bone health and healing. Vitamin D is also essential in injury recovery, as it promotes bone mineralization and remodeling, as well as regulates circulating inflammatory cells and cytokines.[1] Given these data, vitamin D laboratory values are commonly measured in orthopedic surgery patients.[2] Within the arthroplasty realm,

there is a notably high prevalence of vitamin D deficiency among elderly patients with osteoarthritis undergoing total joint arthroplasty (TJA).[3] This finding has also been shown more broadly, with a high proportion of patients with hypovitaminosis D (as high as 62.9%) among patients of all ages undergoing TJA.[4] Thus, it may be important to monitor vitamin D levels in this patient population, as this remains a concern for arthroplasty surgeons and primary care physicians in terms of providing optimal longitudinal patient care.

[a] Harvard Medical School, 25 Shattuck Street, Boston, MA 02115, USA; [b] Department of Orthopaedic Surgery, Brigham and Women's Hospital, 75 Francis Street, Boston, MA 02115, USA
* Corresponding author. 55 Fruit Street, Boston, MA 02114.
E-mail address: Jessica_duggan@hms.harvard.edu

Orthop Clin N Am 55 (2024) 323–332
https://doi.org/10.1016/j.ocl.2024.02.002
0030-5898/24/© 2024 Elsevier Inc. All rights reserved.

Much of the current literature investigating vitamin D levels in arthroplasty patients focuses on the implications of preoperative vitamin D deficiency before undergoing primary total knee arthroplasty (TKA). Preoperative vitamin D deficiency has been associated with longer hospital length of stay and lower functional outcomes following TKA.[5] Specifically, having serum vitamin D levels greater than 20 ng/mL prior to surgery is associated with an increased incidence of postoperative complications following TKA, including postoperative stiffness resulting in manipulation under anesthesia, surgical-site infections resulting in operative management, and prosthesis explantation at 1 year postoperatively.[6] There have also been numerous cardiovascular complications including deep vein thrombosis, myocardial infarction, and cerebrovascular accident, that have been associated with vitamin D deficiency before TKA.[6]

While the literature has historically emphasized patients undergoing primary TKA procedures, the rates of revision TKA are rising worldwide and projected to continue increasing.[7] This is likely due to greater longevity of the population and increased burden of osteoarthritis, leading to a greater number of primary TKA procedures being performed at baseline as well as a greater proportion of patients outliving their prosthetic implants.[7] While there are some widely established risk factors for undergoing revision TKA[8,9]—including demographic (younger age, male sex, Black race), surgical (malalignment, uncemented implants), and institutional (lower volume medical centers)—research on vitamin D status as a risk factor remains ongoing. Kong and colleagues found that patients who received vitamin D supplementation had a lower risk of undergoing revision TKA, and this was true for patients with a periprosthetic joint infection (PJI) and those without any infection.[10] In terms of postoperative outcomes after revision hip and knee arthroplasty, low vitamin D (level <30 ng/mL) was shown to be associated with an increased risk of 90 day complications and PJI requiring additional surgery,[11] which is similar to findings in the primary TKA literature.

Despite the evidence of poorer outcomes following revision TKA in patients with vitamin D deficiency, there is a lack of data investigating long-term postoperative vitamin D levels and supplementation regimens in these patients. Mouli and colleagues proposed that preoperative vitamin D deficiency should be corrected with a loading dose of 50,000 IU weekly for 4 weeks followed by a dose of 2000 IU/day up until TKA.[12] In a randomized control trial, it was found that a single dose of 50,000 IU of vitamin D on the morning of TKA led to no difference in functional Knee Society Scores, Timed Up and Go Test times, or early postoperative complications.[13] Still, these proposals for addressing vitamin D deficiency are limited by lack of quantitative data regarding patients' actual vitamin D levels,[4] and there are no standardized guidelines for management in the postoperative period, especially for patients undergoing revision TKA. This is in contrast to several general surgery domains, in which postoperative vitamin D supplementation has demonstrated improved patient outcomes.[14,15]

Given the paucity of data specific to revision TKA patients, we sought to investigate long-term postoperative vitamin D levels and vitamin D supplementation after revision TKA. The objectives of this study were to evaluate (1) vitamin D levels; (2) the relationship between vitamin D supplementation and vitamin D status; (3) factors related to deficiency, that is, vitamin D levels less than 30 ng/mL; and (4) factors related to vitamin D repletion, that is, becoming sufficient after being deficient, in patients following revision TKA procedures. We hypothesized that there would be a high prevalence of vitamin D deficiency in these patients and that taking supplementation would be associated with both higher vitamin D levels and better ability to achieve repletion.

MATERIALS AND METHODS
Study Design
We performed a retrospective cohort analysis after obtaining approval from the Institutional Review Board (IRB #2022P003414). The analysis included all patients who underwent revision TKA at a single hospital between January 1, 2015 and December 31, 2022, performed by 3 arthroplasty fellowship trained surgeons. Patients were identified through our institutional Research Patient Data Registry. We used the Current Procedural Terminology code 27487 for "revision of total knee arthroplasty, with or without allograft, femoral and entire tibial component."[16] Inclusion criteria for this study were age 18 years and above, history of revision TKA, and documentation of vitamin D laboratory values postoperatively up to 2 years. Patients were excluded from the study if they lacked any postoperative vitamin D laboratory values (n = 29) or died within 2 years of their procedure date (n = 0).

Data Collection
For each patient in the study, we obtained basic demographic information: age, sex assigned at

birth, race, language, ethnicity, and vital status (ie, deceased or not reported as deceased). For each revision TKA procedure performed, we collected the date of surgery (DOS), 25-OH vitamin D (calcidiol) levels preoperatively and postoperatively, and entire patient medication lists. Laboratory results were sorted in reference to the DOS: preoperative (within 90 days prior to surgery) and postoperative (1 month, 3 months, 6 months, 1 year, and 2 years). Although there is varying consensus in the literature regarding the numeric cutoffs for vitamin D deficiency, newer evidence suggests 30 ng/mL as a minimum target vitamin D level for the healthy population.[17,18] Levels of 30 ng/mL and above have shown to be important for achieving optimal effects on metabolism, immunity, and bone health.[19] Therefore, as outlined by the Institute of Medicine,[20] we defined vitamin D sufficiency in this study as 30 ng/mL and above, and deficiency as any level below 30 ng/mL. Medications recorded included any vitamin D products (ergocalciferol/vitamin D2 or cholecalciferol/vitamin D3). The vitamin D supplementation regimens were sorted by dose: low dose (1000 IU and below), medium dose (1001–5000 IU), and high dose (>5000 IU).

Statistical Analysis
Microsoft Excel was used to calculate the following descriptive statistics: item category counts, mean values, and standard deviations. Statistical tests performed for this study include Student's t-test, dependent samples (paired) t-test, chi-squared test, Fisher's exact test, and logistic regression. Logistic regressions were performed to assess potential explanatory effects on the likelihood that a patient will have vitamin D deficiency (vitamin D level <30 ng/mL) and the likelihood that a patient achieved repletion following vitamin D deficiency. All statistical analyses were performed with IBM SPSS software (Armonk, NY, 2021).

RESULTS
Demographics and Medication Regimens
There were a total of 20 patients included in the study (70% female sex, n = 14) who underwent a total of 23 revision TKA procedures. Three patients underwent multiple revisions of the same ipsilateral knee. Eight (40%) patients were between 45 and 64 years old, 8 patients (40%) were between 65 and 79 years old, and 4 (20%) patients were aged 80 years or older. Nineteen (95%) patients identified as White and one (5%) patient identified as Black. Female sex was significantly associated with being prescribed vitamin

D (P = .039). Broken down by supplementation doses, female sex was associated with low and medium dose, while male sex was associated with no supplementation (P = .024). Otherwise, there were no significant group differences in age or race between the supplementation and no supplementation cohorts (Table 1). The average time from primary to revision TKA was 3.89 ± 4.85 years overall. The supplementation group had a longer average time from primary to revision TKA compared to the no supplementation group (4.88 vs 2.48 years), though this was not statistically significant (P = .264).

Thirteen (57%) patients received vitamin D supplementation in the perioperative window of their revision TKA while 10 (43%) patients were not prescribed any vitamin D supplementation. Of those receiving supplementation, 9 (69%) were prescribed the medication prior to surgery and 4 (31%) were prescribed the medication within 14 days postoperatively. Patients were further stratified in terms of their preoperative vitamin D status: 6 (26%) were sufficient preoperatively and received supplementation, 3 (13%) were deficient preoperatively and received supplementation, 3 (13%) were sufficient preoperatively and did not receive supplementation, zero (0%) were deficient preoperatively and did not receive supplementation, and 11 (48%) did not have preoperative laboratory values drawn within 14 days prior to surgery. The average length of follow up with 18.9 ± 8.35 months (range 1–24 months), and the length of follow-up did not differ between supplementation groups (P = .834).

We then separated those who received supplementation into various dose categories. Seven patients (54%) received low dose (1000 IU and below), 3 (23%) received medium dose (1001–5000 IU), and 3 (23%) received high dose (>5000 IU). Regarding the type of supplementation prescribed, 1 (8%) patient was prescribed ergocalciferol (vitamin D2) and 12 (92%) were prescribed cholecalciferol (vitamin D3).

Vitamin D Levels
For all patients in the study, the mean vitamin D levels (measured in ng/mL) were 43.58 ± 27.39 preoperatively before revision TKA, and 34.67 ± 21.60 at 1 month postoperatively, 25.80 ± 9.42 at 3 months, 47.33 ± 14.98 at 6 months, 32.60 ± 16.09 at 1 year, and 38.79 ± 15.42 at 2 years (Table 2). When comparing patients who received supplementation to those who did not, the group receiving supplementation showed higher vitamin D levels preoperatively, and postoperatively at 1 month,

Table 1
Patient demographics

Variables	Category	Prescribed Vitamin D (n = 12)	Not Prescribed Vitamin D (n = 8)	P-value
Sex at birth				P=.039[a]
	Male	2	4	
	Female	10	4	
Age (years)				P=.269
	45–64	6	2	
	65–79	4	4	
	80+	2	2	
Race				P=1.000
	White	11	8	
	Black	1	0	

[a] Statistically significant.

3 months, and 2 years, though these differences were not statistically significant. However, the supplementation group had lower vitamin D levels at 1 year postoperatively when compared to the no supplementation group (25.67 vs 43.00 ng/mL, respectively, P = .095; Table 3).

Next, we stratified patients by preoperative vitamin D status (sufficient preoperatively and deficient preoperatively). In the group of patients who were vitamin D sufficient preoperatively, patients who took supplementation had higher vitamin D levels than patients who did not at the following time points: preoperative, 3 month, and 2 years. Again, the supplementation group demonstrated lower vitamin D levels at 1 year compared to the no supplementation group, though these differences were not significant (Table 4). A subgroup analysis of the patients who were vitamin D deficient preoperatively could not be performed, as all of these patients received supplementation and thus there was no comparison group who did not receive supplementation.

We also assessed the role of vitamin D supplementation on each patient's paired laboratory values, to account for individual trends in vitamin D levels. Interestingly, those who were prescribed supplementation showed significantly lower vitamin D levels postoperatively at 3 months (−9.50 mg/dL on average, P = .033) and 1 year (−19.00 mg/dL on average, P = .042) when compared to baseline. These differences were not seen in the group of patients who did not receive supplementation. Neither group (receiving supplementation or not receiving supplementation) demonstrated significantly different vitamin D levels at the 2 year time point when compared to baseline measurements (Table 5).

We then analyzed the effect of dosing regimens (no supplementation, low dose, medium dose, and high dose supplementation) on patients' vitamin D levels at each time point. When comparing those who did not take supplementation to those prescribed high-dose vitamin D, the high-dose group again showed lower vitamin D levels at the 2 year follow-up compared to the no supplementation group (vitamin D 26.00 ng/mL vs 36.94 ng/mL, P = .045). There were no significant group differences between patients taking no supplementation and those taking low dose or medium dose supplementation. When comparing low-dose vitamin D to high-dose vitamin D regimens, patients taking high-dose supplementation had lower vitamin D levels preoperatively and postoperatively at 1 month, 6 months, 1 year, and

Table 2
Vitamin D laboratory values for entire patient population

Time Point	N	Mean Vitamin D Level (ng/mL)	Standard Deviation
Preoperative	12	43.58	27.39
1 mo post-op	3	34.67	21.60
3 mo post-op	5	25.80	9.42
6 mo post-op	3	47.33	14.98
1 y post-op	10	32.60	16.09
2 y post-op	16	38.79	15.42

Table 3
Vitamin D laboratory values for supplementation and nonsupplementation groups

Time Point	(−) Vitamin D Supplementation		(+) Vitamin D Supplementation		P-value for Difference in Means
	Mean	Standard Deviation	Mean	Standard Deviation	P-value
Preoperative	38.33	12.70	45.33	31.27	0.721
1 mo	12.00	NA	46.00	12.73	0.274
3 mo	22.00	9.90	28.33	10.21	0.542
6 mo	n/a	NA	47.33	14.98	n/a
1 y	43.00	17.49	25.67	11.76	0.095
2 y	36.94	9.16	40.22	19.43	0.688

Abbreviation: NA, not applicable.

2 years; the 2 year time point was the only one to approach statistical significance (vitamin D 48.75 ng/dL in low-dose group compared to 26.00 ng/dL in high-dose group, $P = .056$). There were no significant group differences found between low and medium dose, or between medium and high dose vitamin D.

Vitamin D Deficiency
There were a total of 13 patients with vitamin D deficiency at any time point (57%). Of these 13 patients, 2 (15%) were deficient preoperatively, 10 (77%) were deficient postoperatively, and 1 (8%) was deficient both preoperatively and postoperatively. We found no significant association between vitamin D deficiency and any of the following supplementation variables: presence of vitamin D supplementation (taking vs not taking), timing of supplementation (prescribed preoperatively vs postoperatively), or type of supplementation (ergocalciferol vs cholecalciferol). In terms of dose category (none, low, medium, high), there was a significant association between high-dose vitamin D supplementation and vitamin D deficiency ($P = .045$).

In terms of demographics, we found no association between vitamin D deficiency and patient race or sex at birth. Patients with vitamin D deficiency were significantly younger in age (mean 63.69 ± 9.63 years) compared to vitamin D sufficient patients (mean 72.10 ± 9.46 years, $P = .049$). The logistic regression further demonstrated that patient age was a significant predictor of vitamin D deficiency. Increasing age was associated with lower odds of having vitamin D deficiency at any time (odds ratio $= 0.82$, $P = .046$). Sex, race, and vitamin D supplementation status were not significant predictors of vitamin D deficiency.

Vitamin D Repletion
Of the 13 total patients with vitamin D deficiency, 7 (54%) of them achieved repletion, that is, achieved a vitamin D level of 30 ng/dL or above. Five patients achieved vitamin D repletion while taking supplementation and 2 patients achieved repletion without taking supplementation. Of the 6 patients who did not achieve repletion, half of them were prescribed vitamin D. The average time to repletion was 12.00 ± 7.75 months (range: 3–24 months).

Table 4
Comparison of vitamin D levels in patients who were vitamin D sufficient preoperatively

Time Point	(−) Vitamin D Supplementation	(+) Vitamin D Supplementation	Difference in Means	P-value for Difference in Means
Preoperative	38.33	56.83	18.50	0.392
1 mo	NA	46.00	NA	NA
3 mo	29.00	30.50	1.50	0.942
6 mo	NA	49.50	NA	NA
1 y	47.00	30.00	−17.00	0.336
2 y	38.00	46.25	8.25	0.798

Abbreviation: NA, not applicable.

Table 5
Comparisons of vitamin D levels among no supplementation versus supplementation cohorts

Pairing	(−) Vitamin D Supplementation Difference in Means (Paired)	P-value	(+) Vitamin D Supplementation Difference in Means (Paired)	P-value
Preoperative → 1 mo	NA	NA	5.50	0.816
Preoperative → 3 mo	NA	NA	−9.50	0.033[a]
Preoperative → 6 mo	NA	NA	11.00	0.118
Preoperative → 1 y	8.67	0.142	−19.00	0.042[a]
Preoperative → 2 y			−7.67	0.524
3 mo → 1 y	11.50	0.237	−9.50	0.382
3 mo → 2 y	NA	NA	5.67	0.733
1 y → 2 y	−16.50	0.459	11.00	0.339

Abbreviation: NA, not applicable.
[a] Statistically significant.

We did not find a significant difference in the time required to reach repletion between the supplementation and no supplementation groups. Additionally, there were no significant association between achieving vitamin D repletion and the following supplementation variables: presence of vitamin D supplementation (taking vs not taking), timing of supplementation (prescribed preoperatively vs postoperatively), type of supplementation (ergocalciferol vs cholecalciferol), or dose category (none, low, medium, high). The logistic regression found no significant predictors of achieving vitamin D replete status.

DISCUSSION

It has been well documented that vitamin D plays a vital role in healthy recovery from orthopedic procedures, including fracture fixation and reconstructive procedures.[1,21] Despite this, vitamin D deficiency is quite common among orthopedic surgery patient populations, affecting at least 67% of foot and ankle patients, 85% of spinal fusion patients, and 63% of arthroplasty patients.[22,23] Moreover, hypovitaminosis D has been associated with poorer functional outcomes and increased complication rates following both primary and revision TKA.[5,6,11] Yet, there is no standard of care regarding vitamin D monitoring and supplementation following revision TKA. To our knowledge, this is the first study of patients who underwent revision TKA that quantifies longer term vitamin D levels (from preoperative up to 2 years postoperatively) and vitamin D repletion regimens.

Our principal findings include (1) when comparing overall vitamin D levels, patients taking supplementation showed higher levels preoperatively, and postoperatively at 1 month, 3 months, and 2 years, though these differences were not statistically significant. However, (2) when assessing paired data for each patient, those who were prescribed supplementation showed significantly lower vitamin D levels postoperatively at 3 months and 1 year when compared to their baseline levels. (3) In comparing dose regimens, the high-dose group showed significantly lower vitamin D levels at 2 years compared to the no supplementation group. (4) Over half of the patients were vitamin D deficient for at least one measured time point. Patients with vitamin D deficiency were significantly younger in age when compared to vitamin D sufficient patients. (5) About half of the vitamin D deficient patients achieved repletion, and the average time to repletion was 1 year. Lastly, (6) female sex was significantly associated with low or medium dose regimens, while male sex was associated with no supplementation.

These findings support the need for ongoing vitamin D surveillance during the postoperative course following revision TKA. The majority of patients (77%, n = 10) with vitamin D deficiency in this study became deficient in the postoperative window. The paired patient data also indicated that there was a large decrease in vitamin D levels (by 19.00 mg/dL) from the preoperative to the 1 year postoperative time points in patients who were prescribed supplementation, which was contrary to our hypothesis. This suggests that empiric vitamin D supplementation without close monitoring may not adequately address patients' vitamin D levels. Additionally, the repletion process itself was lengthy, with an average time to repletion of about 1 year postoperatively, and about half of the patients with deficiency did not achieve repletion by the 2 year follow-up. Thus, this supports longer term (ie, beyond 2 years in some circumstances) postoperative vitamin D monitoring to ensure repletion is reached.

The lower levels of vitamin D seen in the group of patients taking high-dose supplementation were unexpected and suggest there may be additional factors at play contributing to lower vitamin D levels. This includes a lack of UVB radiation, nutritional co-deficiencies, obesity, inflammation, and renal disease.[24] Additionally, high-dose vitamin D (eg, 50,000 IU) is often prescribed on a weekly, biweekly, or monthly basis. These dosing intervals may potentially be too infrequent and difficult to consistently maintain (compliance issues), leading to lack of benefit on overall vitamin D levels. This evidence supports the benefits of prescribing low-to-medium vitamin D dose for revision TKA patients, with caution around anticipated medication adherence. That is, patients may be more likely to adhere to a low–medium daily dose than a weekly/monthly high dose. Nonetheless, poor adherence to daily vitamin D supplementation remains a challenge for clinicians, again supporting the role of continued laboratory surveillance.[25]

It was notable that over 40% of all patients in the study became vitamin D deficient in the postoperative time course, which further highlights the importance of continued monitoring and counseling of patients after TKA. Patients should be counseled at postoperative visits on the need to take vitamin D consistently, even if prior levels have been normal, as natural sources of vitamin D (ie, diet, sunlight) may be insufficient for maintaining healthy serum levels.[26] Although the results of this study were likely not powered enough to show quantitative benefits of taking low or medium dose supplementation, national guidelines recommend all people receive daily vitamin D supplementation. The Institute of Medicine recommends 600 IU daily for individuals aged 1 to 70 years and 800 IU for those 71 years and older,[27] while the Bone Health and Osteoporosis Foundation (BHOF) recommends 800 to 1000 IU daily for adults aged 50 years and older.[28] Further studies are warranted to determine whether higher than standard doses would be beneficial for revision TKA patients.

Extending beyond the national guidelines, numerous studies within and beyond orthopedic surgery have proposed supplementation regimens for the perioperative window. Randomized control trials in orthopedic trauma have shown varying outcomes with vitamin D supplementation. Bischoff and colleagues found that a daily dose of 800 IU led to a 10% risk reduction in hip fractures,[29] while others have found that supplementation with 100,000 IU once or 2000 IU daily did not impact long bone fracture union or fracture risk, respectively.[30,31] In other surgical subspecialties, vitamin D supplementation has shown to decrease the risk of severe clinical complications in patients undergoing thyroidectomy (20 IU daily), liver transplant (2500 IU daily), and coronary artery bypass grafting (600,000 IU once).[15,32–34] Guidelines for supplementation following bariatric surgery are variable, ranging from 400 IU daily to 50,000 IU 3 times weekly, but emphasize consistent supplementation in the 2 year postoperative window.[35,36] Despite the lack of standardization per procedure, it is clear that empiric vitamin D supplementation can benefit patients undergoing major surgical procedures.

Interestingly, sex assigned at birth and patient age were demographic factors associated with vitamin D supplementation and deficiency, respectively. In terms of sex, more female patients undergoing revision TKA were prescribed vitamin D when compared to their male counterparts; specifically, female patients were more likely to be prescribed low or medium dose supplementation. Given current evidence that women have lower vitamin D levels than men independent of body mass index,[37] providers may be more likely to prescribe vitamin D to female patients undergoing TKA. However, male sex is a widely established risk factor for needing revision TKA.[8,9] Moreover, in a longitudinal cohort study of nearly 10,000 patients, male sex was shown to be an independent risk factor for postoperative complications after revision TKA.[38] Given these risks, it may be best practice to standardize vitamin D repletion across male and female patients. Regarding patient's age, our study found that increasing age was associated with lower odds of having vitamin D deficiency at any time. This may be due to older patients having taken vitamin D supplementation for a longer period. Additionally, primary care providers may be more cognizant of vitamin D deficiency in their older patients and thus prescribe supplementation more frequently, despite newer evidence suggesting that vitamin D deficiency is quite prevalent among all age groups, including young adults.[39,40]

Clinically, it is important to establish a standard of care for all patients following revision TKA. Although our sample was small, this long-term study provides evidence that vitamin D deficiency is common in revision TKA patients, and thus we should continue long-term laboratory surveillance to ensure these patients achieve repletion. Moreover, low-to-medium dose vitamin D is safe for patients to take, and in fact, likely significantly under-prescribed in the regions of the world farther from the equator.[26] There is very low concern for vitamin D toxicity, which is quite rare and reported to occur after chronic supplementation with at least 40,000 IU daily.[41] Given this risk–benefit profile and the previously outlined national guidelines, it would be reasonable to prescribe 1000 to 5000 IU of cholecalciferol daily to all patients following revision TKA, though additional work is necessary to specify the optimal dose regimen. Further research should also be done to characterize the role of vitamin D supplementation in larger cohorts of patients undergoing revision TKA and the clinical outcomes associated with vitamin D deficiency.

Our study has several limitations. First, the sample size was quite small (n = 20 patients, n = 23 procedures), as 29 patients were excluded due to lack of postoperative vitamin D laboratory values, greatly limiting the power of our analyses. Second, despite being able to access patients' lifetime medications and their date of prescription, quantity, and dosage through review of the patient database, it is unlikely that we captured completely accurate regimens. Patients may take more or less vitamin D than prescribed (eg, missed doses, over the counter supplementations not documented in the medical record) and may consume vitamin D through diet. As with any oral medication, it is difficult to assess patient adherence regularly. Third, although there is literature on implications of vitamin D deficiency after revision TKA, we did not assess clinical or functional patient outcomes in this study. Fourth, this study analyzed patients at a single hospital in New England whose surgeries were done by arthroplasty-trained orthopedic surgeons. Given that high volume medical institutions are a protective factor against needing a revision TKA,[8,9] our results may not be generalizable to community settings. Finally, the diversity in our patient population was limited, with 95% of patients identifying as White race; thus, it would be meaningful to extend this analysis to a more diverse study population.

In conclusion, we found that vitamin D deficiency is common among patients undergoing revision TKA, supporting the need for long-term postoperative vitamin D surveillance. Patients who were prescribed vitamin D did not show improved vitamin D levels. Specifically, taking high-dose vitamin D was associated with vitamin D deficiency at 2 years postoperatively, though we are unable to evaluate patient compliance with various regimens. Younger patient age may be a risk factor for developing vitamin D deficiency after revision TKA. Higher powered studies should be done to further investigate the relationship between patient factors, supplementation regimens, and clinical outcomes with respect to vitamin D levels after revision arthroplasty.

CLINIC CARE POINTS

- Over 50% of patients undergoing revision TKA demonstrated vitamin D deficiency at any time point.

- Daily low-dose cholecalciferol (vitamin D3, 1000 IU or less) was the most common supplementation regimen prescribed to revision TKA patients, which is consistent with recommendations set forth by the Institute of Medicine and the BHOF.

- High-dose vitamin D (often prescribed as 50,000 IU weekly, biweekly, or monthly) was associated with worse vitamin D levels at 2 year follow-up, and may be more difficult for patients to adhere to than a smaller daily dose.

- Female sex was associated with being prescribed vitamin D supplementation, and male sex was associated with not being prescribed vitamin D, despite male sex being a risk factor for both undergoing a revision TKA and having postoperative complications after revision.

- Among patients undergoing revision TKA, younger age was associated with incidence of vitamin D deficiency at any time point.

ACKNOWLEDGMENTS

The first author of this study, Student Doctor J.L. Duggan, is a 4th year medical student at Harvard Medical School and researcher within the Brigham and Women's Hospital Department of Orthopedic Surgery. J.L. Duggan has completed numerous projects within the arthroplasty field, including submission of several abstracts and a study this year (2023) related to vitamin D status of arthroplasty patients. I have personally reviewed this article thoroughly and I am confident in the quality of research and scientific writing produced by J.L. Duggan and the remaining members of our research team.

DISCLOSURE

The authors have no commercial of financial conflicts of interest to disclose in the subject matter of this study.

REFERENCES

1. Gorter EA, Hamdy NAT, Appelman-Dijkstra NM, et al. The role of vitamin D in human fracture healing: a systematic review of the literature. Bone 2014;64: 288–97. https://doi.org/10.1016/j.bone.2014.04.026.

2. Tran EY, Uhl RL, Rosenbaum AJ. Vitamin D in Orthopaedics. JBJS Rev 2017;5(8):e1. https://doi.org/10.2106/JBJS.RVW.16.00084.

3. Jansen J, Haddad F. High prevalence of vitamin D deficiency in elderly patients with advanced osteoarthritis scheduled for total knee replacement associated with poorer preoperative functional state. Ann R Coll Surg Engl 2013;95(8):569–72. https://doi.org/10.1308/rcsann.2013.95.8.569.

4. Brambilla L, Peretti GM, Sirtori P, et al. Outcome of total hip and total knee arthroplasty and vitamin D homeostasis. Br Med Bull 2020;135(1):50–61. https://doi.org/10.1093/bmb/ldaa018.

5. Jansen A, Haddad S. Vitamin D deficiency is associated with longer hospital stay and lower functional outcome after total knee arthroplasty. Acta Orthop Belg 2017;83(4):664–70.

6. Hegde V, Arshi A, Wang C, et al. Preoperative Vitamin D Deficiency Is Associated With Higher Postoperative Complication Rates in Total Knee Arthroplasty. Orthopedics 2018;41(4):e489–95. https://doi.org/10.3928/01477447-20180424-04.

7. Hamilton DF, Howie CR, Burnett R, et al. Dealing with the predicted increase in demand for revision total knee arthroplasty: challenges, risks and opportunities. Bone Jt J 2015;97-B(6):723–8. https://doi.org/10.1302/0301-620x.97b6.35185.

8. Jasper LL, Jones CA, Mollins J, et al. Risk factors for revision of total knee arthroplasty: a scoping review. BMC Musculoskelet Disord 2016;17(1):182. https://doi.org/10.1186/s12891-016-1025-8.

9. Dy CJ, Marx RG, Bozic KJ, et al. Risk Factors for Revision Within 10 Years of Total Knee Arthroplasty. Clin Orthop Relat Res 2014;472(4):1198–207. https://doi.org/10.1007/s11999-013-3416-6.

10. Kong Y, Han M, Lee M, et al. The Association of Calcium and Vitamin D Use With Implant Survival of Total Knee Arthroplasty: A Nationwide Population-Based Cohort Study. J Arthroplasty 2021;36(2):542–9.e3. https://doi.org/10.1016/j.arth.2020.08.003.

11. Traven SA, Chiaramonti AM, Barfield WR, et al. Fewer complications following revision hip and knee arthroplasty in patients with normal vitamin D levels. J Arthroplasty 2017;32(9 Supplement): S193–6. https://doi.org/10.1016/j.arth.2017.02.038.

12. Mouli VH, Schudrowitz N, Carrera CX, et al. High-Dose Vitamin D Supplementation Can Correct Hypovitaminosis D Prior to Total Knee Arthroplasty. J Arthroplasty 2022;37(2):274–8. https://doi.org/10.1016/j.arth.2021.10.016.

13. Weintraub MT, Guntin J, Yang J, et al. Vitamin D3 Supplementation Prior to Total Knee Arthroplasty: A Randomized Controlled Trial. J Arthroplasty 2022. https://doi.org/10.1016/j.arth.2022.08.020. Published online August 19.

14. Alhefdhi A, Mazeh H, Chen H. Role of Postoperative Vitamin D and/or Calcium Routine Supplementation in Preventing Hypocalcemia After Thyroidectomy: A Systematic Review and Meta-Analysis. Oncol 2013; 18(5):533–42. https://doi.org/10.1634/theoncologist.2012-0283.

15. Doi J, Moro A, Fujiki M, et al. Nutrition Support in Liver Transplantation and Postoperative Recovery: The Effects of Vitamin D Level and Vitamin D Supplementation in Liver Transplantation. Nutrients 2020;12(12): 3677. https://doi.org/10.3390/nu12123677.

16. Article - Billing and Coding: Total Knee Arthroplasty (A57685).https://www.cms.gov/medicare-coverage-database/view/article.aspx?articleId=57685. [Accessed 31 October 2023].

17. Bouillon R, Norman A, Lips P. Vitamin D deficiency [8]. N Engl J Med 2007;357:1980–1. https://doi.org/10.1056/NEJMc072359.

18. Munns CF, Shaw N, Kiely M, et al. Global Consensus Recommendations on Prevention and Management of Nutritional Rickets. J Clin Endocrinol Metab 2016;101(2):394–415. https://doi.org/10.1210/jc.2015-2175.

19. Charoenngam N, Holick MF. Immunologic Effects of Vitamin D on Human Health and Disease. Nutrients 2020;12(7):2097. https://doi.org/10.3390/nu12072097.

20. Looker AC, Johnson CL, Lacher DA, et al. Vitamin D status: United States, 2001-2006. NCHS Data Brief 2011;(59):1–8.

21. Moon AS, Boudreau S, Mussell E, et al. Current concepts in vitamin D and orthopaedic surgery. Orthop Traumatol Surg Res 2019;105(2):375–82. https://doi.org/10.1016/j.otsr.2018.12.006.

22. Michelson JD, Charlson MD. Vitamin D Status in an Elective Orthopedic Surgical Population. Foot Ankle Int 2016;37(2):186–91. https://doi.org/10.1177/1071100715609054.

23. Stoker GE, Buchowski JM, Bridwell KH, et al. Preoperative Vitamin D Status of Adults Undergoing Surgical Spinal Fusion. Spine 2013;38(6):507. https://doi.org/10.1097/BRS.0b013e3182739ad1.

24. Cashman KD. Vitamin D Deficiency: Defining, Prevalence, Causes, and Strategies of Addressing. Calcif Tissue Int 2020;106(1):14–29. https://doi.org/10.1007/s00223-019-00559-4.

25. Mager DR, Jackson ST, Hoffmann MR, et al. Vitamin D supplementation and bone health in adults

with diabetic nephropathy: the protocol for a randomized controlled trial. BMC Endocr Disord 2014;14(1):66. https://doi.org/10.1186/1472-6823-14-66.

26. Pludowski P, Holick MF, Grant WB, et al. Vitamin D supplementation guidelines. J Steroid Biochem Mol Biol 2018;175:125–35. https://doi.org/10.1016/j.jsbmb.2017.01.021.

27. Office of Dietary Supplements - Vitamin D.https://ods.od.nih.gov/factsheets/VitaminD-Consumer/. [Accessed 7 May 2023].

28. LeBoff MS, Greenspan SL, Insogna KL, et al. The clinician's guide to prevention and treatment of osteoporosis. Osteoporos Int 2022;33(10):2049–102. https://doi.org/10.1007/s00198-021-05900-y.

29. Bischoff-Ferrari HA, Willett WC, Orav EJ, et al. A Pooled Analysis of Vitamin D Dose Requirements for Fracture Prevention. N Engl J Med 2012;367(1):40–9. https://doi.org/10.1056/NEJMoa1109617.

30. Haines N, Kempton LB, Seymour RB, et al. The effect of a single early high-dose vitamin D supplement on fracture union in patients with hypovitaminosis D: a prospective randomised trial. Bone Jt J 2017;99-B(11):1520–5. https://doi.org/10.1302/0301-620X.99B11.BJJ-2017-0271.R1.

31. LeBoff MS, Chou SH, Ratliff KA, et al. Supplemental Vitamin D and Incident Fractures in Midlife and Older Adults. N Engl J Med 2022;387(4):299–309. https://doi.org/10.1056/NEJMoa2202106.

32. El-Shinawi M, El-Anwar A, Nada M, et al. Oral calcium and vitamin D supplementation after total thyroidectomy. Thyroid Res Pract 2014;11(3):98. https://doi.org/10.4103/0973-0354.138553.

33. Talasaz AH, Salehiomran A, Heidary Z, et al. The effects of vitamin D supplementation on postoperative atrial fibrillation after coronary artery bypass grafting in patients with vitamin D deficiency.

J Card Surg 2022;37(7):2219–24. https://doi.org/10.1111/jocs.16550.

34. Grant C. A vitamin D protocol post-liver transplantation. J Am Assoc Nurse Pract 2017;29(11):658–66. https://doi.org/10.1002/2327-6924.12503.

35. Chakhtoura MT, Nakhoul N, Akl EA, et al. Guidelines on vitamin D replacement in bariatric surgery: Identification and systematic appraisal. Metabolism 2016;65(4):586–97. https://doi.org/10.1016/j.metabol.2015.12.013.

36. Lanzarini E, Nogués X, Goday A, et al. High-Dose Vitamin D Supplementation is Necessary After Bariatric Surgery: A Prospective 2-Year Follow-up Study. Obes Surg 2015;25(9):1633–8. https://doi.org/10.1007/s11695-015-1572-3.

37. Muscogiuri G, Barrea L, Somma CD, et al. Sex Differences of Vitamin D Status across BMI Classes: An Observational Prospective Cohort Study. Nutrients 2019;11(12):3034. https://doi.org/10.3390/nu11123034.

38. Gu A, Wei C, Bernstein SA, et al. The Impact of Gender on Postoperative Complications after Revision Total Knee Arthroplasty. J Knee Surg 2020;33(4):387–93. https://doi.org/10.1055/s-0039-1677820.

39. Palacios C, Gonzalez L. Is vitamin D deficiency a major global public health problem? J Steroid Biochem Mol Biol 2014;144:138–45. https://doi.org/10.1016/j.jsbmb.2013.11.003.

40. AlQuaiz AM, Kazi A, Fouda M, et al. Age and gender differences in the prevalence and correlates of vitamin D deficiency. Arch Osteoporos 2018;13(1):49. https://doi.org/10.1007/s11657-018-0461-5.

41. Alshahrani F, Aljohani N. Vitamin D: Deficiency, Sufficiency and Toxicity. Nutrients 2013;5(9):3605–16. https://doi.org/10.3390/nu5093605.

Cementless Total Knee Arthroplasty
Is it Safe in Demineralized Bone?

Christopher Deans, MD[a,*], Bradford Zitsch, MD[a],
Beau J. Kildow, MD[a], Kevin L. Garvin, MD[a]

KEYWORDS

- Arthroplasty • Total knee arthroplasty • Cementless total knee • Demineralized bone
- Osteoporosis

KEY POINTS

- Aseptic loosening is one of the most common indications for revision total knee arthroplasty today.
- Advances in cementless total knee implant design and technology have resulted in expanding indications, including in older patients and those with decreased bone mineral density.
- Cementless total knees in decreased bone mineral density can expect migration in the first 6 to 12 months, with high risk of failed ongrowth thereafter.
- Early-term outcomes of contemporary cementless total knee arthroplasty in patients with decreased bone mineral density are mixed, and long-term outcomes not yet known.
- Antiresorptive medications may demonstrate clinical benefit in early-term outcomes; however, the use is associated with higher long-term rate of periprosthetic fracture.

INTRODUCTION

Total knee arthroplasty (TKA) has been performed for over 50 years, with first successful designs and procedures being developed and performed as early as the 1970s. Today, it is the preferred treatment for end-stage osteoarthritis (OA) with the goal to create a painless and functional knee that would survive many years. The volume of procedures being performed is expanded rapidly. Approximately 1.3 million TKAs were performed in the United States in 2020, with future projections of growth to 3.5 million TKAs by 2030.[1]

Cemented TKA have well-established long-term functional outcomes and excellent survivorship, with up to 95% survivorship at minimum 10 years.[2–4] However, with patients living longer, increasing utilization of TKA for younger and more active patients, and low long-term wear

rates of polyethylene, concerns have been raised about long-term durability of cemented TKAs. Several studies have shown moderate rates of aseptic fixation failure at either the bone–cement interface or cement–implant interface.[5,6] In addition, according to the American Joint Replacement Registry (AJRR) Annual Report 2020, cementless TKA in male patients younger than 65 years has shown significantly less revisions than cemented TKA.[7]

As a result, although cementation remains the most commonly used fixation for primary TKA, it is on the decline in the United States and in many other countries. In a survey of current practice trends among members of the American Association of Hip and Knee Surgeons, over 70% of surgeons reported always using cemented fixation in primary TKA in 2018, decreasing to 41% in 2022.[8] In comparison, surgeons using cementless fixation in select cases were reported 27%,

[a] Department of Orthopaedic Surgery and Rehabilitation, University of Nebraska Medical Center, 985640 Nebraska Medical Center, Omaha, NE 68198, USA
* Corresponding author.
E-mail address: christopher.deans@unmc.edu

Orthop Clin N Am 55 (2024) 333–343
https://doi.org/10.1016/j.ocl.2024.02.003

42%, and 61% in 2018, 2020, and 2022, respectively.[8] The AJRR showed cementless fixation has been steadily increasing, from 1.9% of all primary TKAs in 2012 to 18.8% in 2021.[9] The Swedish Knee Arthroplasty Registry (SKAR) noted an increase in cementless TKA from 2.4% in 2010 to 9.1% in 2021, while the National Joint Registry of the England, Wales, Northern Ireland, and the Isle of Man reports a decrease in use of cementless TKA from 5.3% in 2010 to 2.2% in 2021, respectively.[10,11]

Advancements in implant coating and design have resulted in expanding indications for cementless TKA; however, there is particular concern in patients with decreased bone mineral density (BMD).[12–14] Critics of cementless implants in this patient population cite the potential increase in periprosthetic fracture rates, aseptic loosening, failed in-growth, and reduced long-term implant survival compared to cemented counterparts.[15–19] This is particularly relevant considering the prevalence of diagnosed or undiagnosed osteoporosis and osteopenia in total joint arthroplasty (TJA) populations, with reported pooled prevalence up to 64%.[20]

Concern exists due to the greater volume of cementless TKA being performed in a population at risk for osteoporosis and metabolic bone disease. It is crucial to gain understanding of the prevalence and etiology of osteoporosis and osteopenia in the TKA population, how this may affect our utilization of cementless total knees, the survivorship of cementless TKA in this population, the role of bone-modifying agents and other medications may play, and considerations regarding indications and technique for cementless TKA. The purpose of this study is to review current literature and expert opinion on such topics.

OSTEOPOROSIS: AN OVERVIEW

Osteoporosis is common in older adults undergoing arthroplasty and may likely be a risk factor for aseptic loosening, the second most common cause of revision after TKA.[21,22] A previous US study reported a 25% prevalence of osteoporosis in postmenopausal women undergoing total hip arthroplasty (THA).[23] A recent meta-analysis found the prevalence of osteoporosis and osteopenia in TJA patients to be 24.8% and 38.5%, respectively. The prevalence of osteoporosis in males, females, and postmenopausal females were 5.5%, 29.0%, and 38.3%, respectively.[20] More specific to the US population, a 2019 study of 200 consecutive adults undergoing TJA reported that 33% of those who underwent dual-energy X-ray absorptiometry testing prior to surgery were diagnosed with osteoporosis. One-quarter of the entire study cohort met criteria to receive osteoporosis medications, while only 5% received therapy preoperatively or postoperatively.[24] Not only is it likely that the prevalence of osteopenia and osteoporosis in TKA patients is underestimated, but also the appropriate treatment is grossly underprovided.

Osteoporosis is a disease characterized by low bone density, caused by a complex interaction among local and systemic regulators of bone cell function (**Box 1**). Normal bone remodeling is performed in bone multicellular units (BMUs), composed hematopoietic precursors to osteoclasts and immature mesenchymal precursors to osteoblasts, on the surface of trabecular bone or within Haversian systems of cortical bone. These cells are directed or influenced by thousands of aforementioned local or systemic molecules in a complex interplay between genetics, hormones, vitamins and minerals, signals and receptors, and so forth. Generally, skeletal fragility may be the result of (1) failure of bony development to optimal mass and strength during peak growth, (2) excessive bone resorption, or (3) an inadequate bone reformation response to increased bony resorption during remodeling.[25] Any one of these or a complex interaction of multiple results in decrease of bone mass and microarchitectural deterioration of skeletal structure. As bone remodeling occurs on bone surfaces and trabecular bone is fashioned with far more surface area than cortical bone, more remodeling sites per unit volume occurs in trabecular bone than cortical bone. As a result,

---

Box 1
Changes in osteoporosis

Osseous Structural Changes in Osteoporosis[70]

Thinner, more cavernous trabecular cancellous bone.

Cortical thinning with trabecularization of endocortical bony surface.

Increased porous size and number in cortical bone.

Decreased mineralization of trabecular and cortical bone.

Greater spatial distributions of calcium and other bone minerals.

Decreased cross-linking of bone collagen matrix.

Decreased noncollagenous protein mass.

a greater proportion of trabecular bone is turned over, and in the presence of osteoporosis, more trabecular bone is lost with each remodel causing deep resorptive cavities and loss of trabecular plates (trabecular thinning).[26]

BMD is a surrogate marker for bone strength. In reality, specific determinants such as bone geometry, cortical thickness and porosity, trabecular bone architecture, and bone tissue quality all contribute to structure strength and stability. With negative balance at the BMU, this bony structure is expected to display thinner, more cavernous trabeculae, remodeling of the endocortical surface resulting in cortical thinning, and to decrease in trabecular and cortical bone mineralization.[26] These structure and molecular changes are key to concerns that have arisen for the use of cementless implants in TKA.

CEMENTLESS TOTAL KNEE MATERIAL AND DESIGN

Early cementless TKA experience was of little success compared to cemented TKA in long-term outcomes. Failure was most often due to failed on-growth of the tibial, patellar failure or fracture, and few femoral component fractures.[27,28]

Cementless patellar resurfacing most commonly failed due to patellar maltracking, increasing incidence of component fracture, failed on-growth or aseptic loosening, or osteolysis and contributed to a revision rate of up to 56%.[29–31] When the patella failed, removal and revision of the patellar component resulted in catastrophic bone loss or disruption of the extensor mechanism, oftentimes severely impacting postoperative outcomes.[32,33] Design modifications in response to these complications included improving femoral design and introduction of mobile-bearing knees for patellar tracking and modifications of the cementless patellar backside design in attempts to minimize bone loss while maximizing stability.[34,35] Additionally, many continue to cement patellar components with cementless tibial and femoral implants. It is noteworthy that the utility of patellar resurfacing remains a debated topic among surgeons today.[36,37]

Another common failure mechanism in early-generation implants was failed on-growth or aseptic loosening of the tibial components.[27,28,38,39] This was due to poor initial implant rotational and axial fixation and stability, resulting in greater micromotion than allowable for osteogenesis. Modern implants designers have sought to mitigate this with improved keel material and design, porous in-growth surfaces, and additive bioactive materials. Modern keels are most commonly titanium, with better coating in the form of 3 dimensional porous shape that is similar to bone in porosity and texture. This porosity provides significantly improved surface roughness and stability.[38,40] Additionally, implementation of hydroxyapatite coating presents a bioactive material to further enhance osteogenesis and in-growth.[41–43]

POROUS IMPLANT INTERACTION WITH BONE

Various factors contribute to the interaction between implant and bone and are important in understanding how to enhance success of cementless implants: (1) the physical properties and biologic activity of the bone, (2) the mechanical interaction between implant and bone, and (3) the properties and design of the biomaterials. Each of these factors must be satisfied in order to optimize implant osseointegration in cementless TKA.

In the ideal setting, the porous titanium implant with 3 dimensional open, interconnected macropores and micropores and potentially, additive bioactive coating is surgically implanted in an environment of primary implant stability and low micromotion, as well as high osseous biologic potential. Maximization of porous implant to bone contact is achieved, with less than 0.3 to 0.5 mm between bone and implant over the majority of the implant–bone interface.[44] Stimulated by a complex interaction of hormones, cytokines, protein, and other signaling molecules, osteoblasts penetrate into the implant pores with sufficient nutrient supply. Subsequently, cell attachment and vascular proliferation are achieved, providing a strong and durable implant–bone interface. Alteration in any of the 3 factors—bone biology, mechanical stability, and biomaterial properties—could lead to a failure of osseous in-growth and development of a nondurable fibrous union.[45–50]

Little data exist in regard to the amount of bone in-growth expected in cementless TKA or needed to achieve adequate long-term fixation. In canine models, Turner and colleagues reported 40% to 90% in-growth to be adequate; however, in retrieval studies, they described less than 30% bony in-growth in what they determined to be clinically well-functioning knees.[51] It is notable that this canine model was utilizing implant technology that has since been improved.

Tibial components of cemented and cementless TKA have been shown to migrate during their initial postoperative period, followed by increased stabilization.[52–56] Greater migration of components, often expressed as maximum total point migration (MTPM), in the early postoperative period has been shown to be closely related to mechanical loosening of implants.[57,58] High preoperative BMD has been shown to result in less MTPM, while lower preoperative BMD indicates a higher MTPM.[59,60] Pijls and colleagues identified a threshold of 0.54 mm MTPM after 1 year as acceptable for implant survival after 5 years, while an MTPM of 1.6 mm after 1 year was unacceptable. Any migration between years 1 and 3 is closely associated with implant failure.[60] Biomechanical studies from 30 years ago appropriately stressed that the quality of tibial metaphyseal bone is a critical parameter for the fixation of the tibial component.[61] While we do not yet know the allowable parameters for BMD and micromotion, it is apparent that maximizing BMD and minimizing micromotion are important in successful osseointegration of cementless implants.

EFFECT OF MEDICATIONS ON DEMINERALIZED BONE

As aforementioned, a relatively high percentage of patients awaiting TJA have low BMD, while only a small fraction receives treatment to address their bone disease. Most of the literature to support pharmacologic therapy in patients with low BMD is an effort to mitigate future fracture risk, wherein initiation of therapy is often based on an individual's history of risk of fracture in the short and long terms. In regard to TJA and cementless total knee design, studies have clearly shown correlation between preoperative BMD, component migration, and subsequent risk of mechanical loosening.[57–60] Yet, the indications in which pharmacologic therapy is indicated in patients undergoing elective TJA are not clearly defined. Medications to treat osteoporosis are categorized as either antiresorptive or anabolic. Antiresorptive medications primarily decrease the rate of bone resorption, while anabolic medications increase bone formation more than bone resorption.[62]

Antiresorptive agents are often the first-line medication for pharmacologic treatment of low BMD. Bisphosphonate, the most commonly prescribed antiresorptive agent, was first introduced in the 1990s and has become the most widely used drug for treatment of osteoporosis. Mechanistically, bisphosphonates bind to hydroxyapatite in bone, particularly at sites of active bone remodeling, and reduce the activity of bone-resorbing osteoclasts.[63–68] Shortly after initiation of therapy, the production of new BMUs decreases which allows BMUs at various stages in the remodeling cycle complete the remodeling process by depositing a volume of new bone that reduces the depth of the excavated site.[69] This newly deposited bone can then undergo primary and slower secondary mineralization, thereby reducing cortical porosity, increasing trabecular mineralization and homogeneity effectively reducing the risk of microdamage, and increasing the BMD.[69,70] Other approved antiresorptive treatment options exist such as estrogen agonists/antagonists, estrogens, calcitonin, and denosumab are commonly used second line to bisphosphonates in the pharmacologic treatment of osteoporosis, and their discussion is out of the scope of this review.

Teriparatide, a recombinant human parathyroid hormone (PTH) analog, is the first anabolic treatment approved for osteoporosis.[62] It mimics the physiologic actions of PTH in stimulating new bone formation on the surface of bone by stimulating osteoblastic activity when given intermittently at small doses.[71] The anabolic effects of (intermittent) PTH are mediated by upregulation of several pro-osteoblastogenic growth factors and subsequent osteoanabolic signaling pathways ultimately necessary for differentiation of osteoblasts.[72–74] This ultimately leads to new growth of trabecular and cortical bone, which stands in contrast both mechanistically and effective result on bone microstructure.

Preserving the periprosthetic bone mass to improve the survival of TKA has been an important subject, particularly with respect to cementless fixation. Following TKA, periprosthetic BMD changes secondary to alteration in the mechanical loads that the knee sees following alignment correction and implantation of a prosthesis, with several studies demonstrating decreased periprosthetic BMD following TKA.[75–78] A meta-analysis by Lin and colleagues found that patients who were started on bisphosphonates at the time of TJA or just thereafter had significantly higher BMD up to 10 years postoperatively.[79] However, most trials in this meta-analysis were in regard to THA with only 2 concerning TKAs. As such, their group performed another meta-analysis of the same methodology in 2018 evaluating trials involving TKA. In 5 randomized controlled trials of 188 total patients, they found that patients who were initiated on bisphosphonates after TKA demonstrated significantly higher BMD in the proximal tibial metaphysis and distal femur than control group at 3, 6, and 12 months postoperatively.[36]

The clinical implications of this in regard to long-term outcomes have also been explored. Several studies have demonstrated that the increase in BMD supports implant fixation and can contribute to a reciprocal reduction in revision rates out to 5 years in patients who are initiated on antiresorptive therapy after undergoing TJA.[80,81] Khatod and colleagues performed a retrospective review of a large database, finding significantly lower risk of aseptic revision and all-cause revision in THA patients taking bisphosphonates.[80] Namba and colleagues reviewed over 34,000 primary TKA patients in the Kaiser Permanente Southern California registry, with nearly 7000 of these patients taking bisphosphonates. They found that the overall aseptic revision rate was lower in the bisphosphonate group (0.5%) than the nonbisphosphonate group (1.6%) at a mean follow-up of 3.7 years.[82] They also found that this effect was age-independent—equally as efficacious for patients less than 65 years as patients ≥ 65 years. Another meta-analysis reviewed 331,660 TKA patients with follow-up between 4 and 14 years, finding a 1.4% all-cause revision rate for bisphosphonate users, compared to 2.9% for nonbisphospohonate users.[81] Lastly, in a case–control meta-analysis of approximately 1500 bisphosphonate users matched to nearly 9000 nonbisphosphonate users, the use of bisphosphonates was correlated with lower revision rate at a median follow-up of 2.61 years (1.73% vs 4.45%, respectively).[83] Notably, these studies contained significantly more cemented TKA patients than cementless TKA patients, and none of them stratified the 2 groups in their reporting.

There are also risks of taking antiresorptive agents after TJA. Prolonged use of bisphosphonates (>5 years) for treatment of osteoporosis has been associated with atypical femur fractures.[84] Khatod and colleagues in their retrospective review of over 12,000 patients after THA found that although there was a lower risk of all-cause revision, there was a significantly higher risk of periprosthetic fracture (Hazard Ratio [HR] 19.2), particularly in those younger than 65 years.[80] Multiple other studies corroborated this finding, reporting increased risk of periprosthetic fractures, especially in younger patients, and this must be taken into consideration when considering bisphosphonate use in TJA.[80,82,83]

It would seem that there is no refuting that bisphosphonates do indeed increase BMD after TKA. Literature also seems to suggest that there may be a benefit to bisphosphonate use in

patients aged 65 years or more in the early postoperative period. However, prolonged use of bisphosphonates and use in younger patients seem to carry with it significant increased risk of periprosthetic fracture. In addition, there are paucity of data on the effects of antiresorptive medications in cementless TKA. Physicians must take these considerations into account when making decisions about antiresorptive medications in the perioperative period.

CEMENTLESS TOTAL KNEE OUTCOMES IN DEMINERALIZED BONE

As implant design and techniques have improved with advancements as aforementioned, there has been renewed interest in cementless fixation, expanding indications, and direct comparison of fixation techniques in the literature. Traditionally, cementless TKA have exhibited worse implant survivorship than cemented equivalents; however, many recent studies have looked at clinical and radiographic outcomes between cemented and cementless TKA at early-to-mid-term follow-up. Nam and colleagues showed no difference in the Knee Society Score (KSS), overall satisfaction, or subsidence and/or progressive radiolucent lines between the cemented and cementless TKAs of the same modern design at 2 year follow-up.[85] A 2021 systemic review and meta-analysis by Liu and colleagues found similar results. In comparison of cemented and cementless TKA with 2 to 16 year follow-up, they found no significant difference in KSSs or range of motion between the 2 groups. Moreover, they found no difference in survivorship with 4.9% all-cause revision in the cementless group and 4% all-cause revision in the cemented group at a minimum of 2 years, with 2.4% and 2.9% (P = .88) undergoing revision for aseptic loosening in the cementless and cemented groups, respectively.[86] Other meta-analyses have found similar results with no significant difference in all-cause or aseptic survivorship between cementless and cemented components.[12,13,87,88]

While these studies broadly provide insight into cemented versus cementless TKA, they do not account for or specifically stratify these outcomes with regard to patients with demineralized bone and few studies have directly compared cemented versus cementless fixation for patients undergoing TKA with low BMD. Therbo and colleagues evaluated 106 uncemented TKAs performed between 1986 and 1991. At 9 to 14 years of follow-up, there was an 11.3% revision rate for aseptic loosening, but they found that low trabecular bone quality, measured as the preoperative bone mineral content of the proximal tibia, was not a predictor for later revision surgery following uncemented TKA.[89] Similarly, Dixon and colleagues prospectively studied 559 patients (of whom 135 were >75 years) undergoing TKA with an HA-coated uncemented implant and found no functional or clinical outcome differences between the greater than 75 year age group and any other of the age groups.[90] More recently, Gibbons and colleagues and Goh and colleagues each similarly found that the theoretic risks of cementless fixation in an advanced age group, both men and women, were not realized. Gibbons and colleagues found 4 of 1000 cementless TKA in women over 75 years with subsidence in the first year, with no cases requiring revision.[91] Goh and colleagues reported a 7 year aseptic survival (99.4% cemented, 100% cementless) in 120 cementless total knees in patients greater than 75 years (range, 75–92).[92]

In contrast, registry data at present report higher revision rates in cementless TKA.[2–4,93] The NJR for England, Wales, and Northern Ireland reports revision rates in number of revisions per 1000 prosthesis-years. The all-cause and lysis or aseptic loosening rates reported for cemented TKA are 3.84 and 1.05, compared to uncemented TKA 4.59 and 1.6, respectively.[2] Similarly, over the last 10 year time period, the SKAR reported significantly higher risk of revision in cementless TKA compared to cemented TKA.[10] A 2022 meta-analysis of Sweden (SKAR), Australia (AOANJRR), and Kaiser Permanente (KPJRR) registries reported a lower risk of revision at 5 and 15 years with cement fixation compared to cementless.[94] It is to be noted that these registry data include all patient ages and specifics, as greater granularity is not available.

Overall, early-to-mid-term data do suggest that recent advances in cementless prostheses could confer a biological fixation that mitigates the risks of decreased bone remodeling and osseointegration associated with patients with decreased BMD. However, this is in opposition to longer term outcomes reported via registry data. More direct comparisons of patients with known osteoporosis undergoing cementless total knee fixation are needed.

TECHNICAL CONSIDERATIONS

Arguably a principal cause for poor outcomes in cementless knee arthroplasty is poor surgical technique, and many technical considerations exist in order to maximize initial implant stability, long-term osseointegration, and subsequent clinical success when performing cementless TKA (Box 2). Bony preparation of both the femur and tibia is critically important, in that accurate and planar cuts of the femur and tibia are essential to avoid slight irregularities which can be a source of poor initial fixation with a cementless implant, ultimately risking mechanical failure.[95] Executing an accurate planar cut of the distal femur must be done with great attention as any error will be magnified in the chamfer and condylar cuts due to the linked planar cuts through the four-in-one cutting guide. Differential hardness is frequently encountered such that sclerotic bone is found on the medial or lateral femoral condyle depending on the patient's coronal plane alignment. This can be seen on both the femoral and tibial sides and attention must be given to the tendency of the saw blade to skive. Sclerotic bone may further generate excessive heat, which may lead to thermal necrosis. Saw blade irrigation may reduce thermal effects, along with some investigators suggesting a new saw blade for each cut.[96] Tibial resection depth must also be scrutinized and should be minimized to utilize the thinnest polyethylene when possible[97]; however, under-resecting can leave excessively hard subchondral bone resulting in a suboptimal bleeding bone for noncemented fixation, whereas a deeper, over-resection into soft metaphyseal bone can significantly increase the proximal tibial strain.[96,98]

Box 2
Technical considerations

Author's Recommended Technical Considerations in Cementless TKA

Precise, flat femoral and tibial cuts.

Minimize heat generation (irrigation during cuts, new saw blade for each cut, and so forth).

Maximize implant surface area contact to bone.

Skim cut tibia to allow sclerotic and cortical rim support.

Bone slurry at implant–bone interface during implantation.

Minimize polyethylene constraint. If greater constraint than posterior stabilized required, consider cementation.

Mechanical alignment versus restricted kinematic alignment.

When choosing the appropriate tibial component size, it is important to err on the side of maximizing cortical coverage. Undersized tibial components have the relative lack of cortical support and have been shown that results in poorer fixation, a higher degree of continuous migration, and increased subsidence and posterior tilt.[99]

The question of whether systematic mechanical alignment versus kinematic alignment (KA) as the ideal alignment method in TKA has been debated by orthopedic surgeons for quite some time, with no ideal consensus formed. With respect to uncemented total knees, it is feared that KA nonneutral alignment may jeopardize primary and/or secondary uncemented TKA implant fixation due to compartmental overload and tibial component loosening.[100] However, some data exist to suggest that restricted KA allows for adequate secondary fixation with low (0%) revision rates for aseptic loosening in medium-term follow-up.[101] More robust data are needed to make more definitive conclusions in this regard; further, stratifying results based on patients with low BMD undergoing cementless TKA with respect to alignment method has not been done to the authors' knowledge.

SUMMARY

Cementless TKA indications have been expanding rapidly, including utilization in patients with poor BMD secondary to glucocorticoid use, osteoporosis, smoking, or other causes. There are mixed results reported in early-, mid-, and long-term outcome studies. Surgeons should entertain a healthy skepticism for cementless TKA utilization in populations with decreased BMD, particularly in the elderly given such strong outcomes of long-term cemented TKA. In younger and more active patients, contemporary cementless TKA may provide more durable and long-lasting biologic fixation, even in decreased BMD. Open communication with patients regarding the risk and benefit profile is of utmost importance. Longer term outcomes studies and direct comparisons in patients with decreased BMD are needed.

CLINICS CARE POINTS

- As aseptic loosening is one of the most common failure mechanisms in modern TKA, it is recommended to follow strict indications for cementless TKA.

- To maximize success of cementless TKA, meticulous surgical technique is required. It is recommended that conversion to cemented TKA be performed with any concern for bone quality intra-operatively.
- In the absence of clear failure, cementless implants may be monitored with serial radiographs for 6 to 12 months. After that time, intervention is recommended.
- The use of antiresorptive medications may have a clinical role in cementless TKA; however, their use is associated with higher periprosthetic fracture risk and a thorough understanding of appropriate patient monitoring and risk profile is recommended.

DISCLOSURE

The authors have nothing to disclose.

REFERENCES

1. Kurtz SM, Ong KL, Lau E, et al. Impact of the economic downturn on total joint replacement demand in the United States: updated projections to 2021. J Bone Joint Surg Am 2014;96(8):624–30.
2. National Joint Registry. National joint Registry for England, Wales, and Northern Ireland; 17th annual report. 2020. Available at: https://reports.njrcentre.org.uk/Portals/0/PDFdownloads/NJR%2017th%20Annual%20Report%202020.pdf. [Accessed 14 January 2021].
3. New Zealand Orthopaedic Association. The New Zealand joint registry ten year report, January 1999 to December 2008. 2008. Available at: https://nzoa.org.nz/sys-tem/files/NJR%2010%20Year%20Report.pdf. [Accessed 14 January 2021].
4. Australian Orthopaedic Association. National joint replacement registry annual reports. 2020. Available at: https://aoanjrr.sahmri.com/en_GB/annual-reports-2020. [Accessed 14 January 2021].
5. Kutzner I, Hallan G, Høl PJ, et al. Early aseptic loosening of a mobile-bearing total knee replacement. Acta Orthop 2018;89(1):77–83.
6. Arsoy D, Pagnano MW, Lewallen DG, et al. Aseptic Tibial Debonding as a Cause of Early Failure in a Modern Total Knee Arthroplasty Design. Clin Orthop Relat Res 2013;471(1):94–101.
7. American Joint Replacement Registry (AJRR). Annual Report. 2020. Available at: https://www.aaos.org/globalassets/registries/2020-aaos-ajrr-annual-report-preview_final.pdf. [Accessed 5 September 2022].
8. Abdel MP, Carender CN, Berry DJ. Current Practice Trends in Primary Hip and Knee Arthroplasties Among Members of the American Association of

Hip and Knee Surgeons. J Arthroplasty 2023;38(10): 1921–7.e3.

9. Siddiqi A, Levine BR, Springer BD. Highlights of the 2021 American Joint Replacement Registry Annual Report. Arthroplast Today 2022;13:205–7.

10. Swedish Arthroplasty Register (SAR). 2021. Available at: https://sar.registercentrum.se/. [Accessed 26 October 2023].

11. National Joint Registry of England, Wales, Northern Ireland, and the Isle of Man (NJR). 2021. Available at: https://www.njrcentre.org.uk/. [Accessed 23 October 2023].

12. Zhou K, Yu H, Li J, et al. No difference in implant survivorship and clinical outcomes between full-cementless and full-cemented fixation in primary total knee arthroplasty: A systematic review and meta-analysis. Int J Surg 2018;53:312–9.

13. Salem HS, Tarazi JM, Ehiorobo JO, et al. Cement-less Fixation for Total Knee Arthroplasty in Various Patient Populations: A Literature Review. J Knee Surg 2020;33(9):848–55.

14. Mont MA, Gwam C, Newman JM, et al. Outcomes of a newer-generation cementless total knee arthroplasty design in patients less than 50 years of age. Ann Transl Med 2017;5(Suppl 3):S24.

15. Liddle AD, Pandit H, O'Brien S, et al. Cementless fixation in Oxford unicompartmental knee replacement: a multicentre study of 1000 knees. Bone Joint Lett J 2013;95-B(2):181–7.

16. Campbell MD, Duffy GP, Trousdale RT. Femoral component failure in hybrid total knee arthroplasty. Clin Orthop Relat Res 1998;356:58–65.

17. Whiteside LA. Effect of porous-coating configuration on tibial osteolysis after total knee arthroplasty. Clin Orthop Relat Res 1995;321:92–7.

18. Cloke DJ, Khatri M, Pinder IM, et al. 284 press-fit Kinemax total knee arthroplasties followed for 10 years: poor survival of uncemented prostheses. Acta Orthop 2008;79(1):28–33.

19. Gandhi R, Tsvetkov D, Davey JR, et al. Survival and clinical function of cemented and uncemented prostheses in total knee replacement: a meta-analysis. J Bone Joint Surg Br 2009;91(7):889–95.

20. Xiao PL, Hsu CJ, Ma YG, et al. Prevalence and treatment rate of osteoporosis in patients undergoing total knee and hip arthroplasty: a systematic review and meta-analysis. Arch Osteoporos 2022;17(1):16.

21. Bozic KJ, Kurtz SM, Lau E, et al. The epidemiology of revision total hip arthroplasty in the United States. J Bone Joint Surg Am 2009;91(1):128–33.

22. Bozic KJ, Kurtz SM, Lau E, et al. The epidemiology of revision total knee arthroplasty in the United States. Clin Orthop Relat Res 2010;468(1):45–51.

23. Glowacki J, Hurwitz S, Thornhill TS, et al. Osteoporosis and vitamin-D deficiency among postmenopausal women with osteoarthritis undergoing

total hip arthroplasty. J Bone Joint Surg Am 2003; 85(12):2371–7.

24. Bernatz JT, Brooks AE, Squire MW, et al. Osteoporosis Is Common and Undertreated Prior to Total Joint Arthroplasty. J Arthroplasty 2019;34(7): 1347–53.

25. Raisz LG. Pathogenesis of osteoporosis: concepts, conflicts, and prospects. J Clin Invest 2005; 115(12):3318–25.

26. Parfitt AM, Mathews CH, Villanueva AR, et al. Relationships between surface, volume, and thickness of iliac trabecular bone in aging and in osteoporosis. Implications for the microanatomic and cellular mechanisms of bone loss. J Clin Invest 1983;72(4):1396–409.

27. Peters PC, Engh GA, Dwyer KA, et al. Osteolysis after total knee arthroplasty without cement. J Bone Joint Surg Am 1992;74(6):864–76.

28. Berger RA, Lyon JH, Jacobs JJ, et al. Problems with cementless total knee arthroplasty at 11 years followup. Clin Orthop Relat Res 2001;392:196–207.

29. Healy WL, Wasilewski SA, Takei R, et al. Patellofemoral complications following total knee arthroplasty. Correlation with implant design and patient risk factors. J Arthroplasty 1995;10(2):197–201.

30. Barrack RL, Wolfe MW. Patellar resurfacing in total knee arthroplasty. J Am Acad Orthop Surg 2000; 8(2):75–82.

31. Castro FP, Chimento G, Munn BG, et al. An analysis of Food and Drug Administration medical device reports relating to total joint components. J Arthroplasty 1997;12(7):765–71.

32. Brick GW, Scott RD. The patellofemoral component of total knee arthroplasty. Clin Orthop Relat Res 1988;231:163–78.

33. Dennis DA. Removal of well-fixed cementless metal-backed patellar components. J Arthroplasty 1992;7(2):217–20.

34. Kraay MJ, Darr OJ, Salata MJ, et al. Outcome of metal-backed cementless patellar components: the effect of implant design. Clin Orthop Relat Res 2001;392:239–44.

35. Buechel FF. Long-term followup after mobile-bearing total knee replacement. Clin Orthop Relat Res 2002;404:40–50.

36. Eiel ES, Donnelly P, Chen AF, et al. Outcomes and Survivorships of Total Knee Arthroplasty Comparing Resurfaced and Unresurfaced Patellae. J Arthroplasty 2023;38(7 S2):S227–32.

37. Schmidt GJ, Farooq H, Deckard ER, et al. Selective Patella Resurfacing in Contemporary Cruciate Retaining and Substituting Total Knee Arthroplasty: A Matched Cohort Analysis. J Arthroplasty 2023; 38(3):491–6.

38. Bhimji S, Meneghini RM. Micromotion of cementless tibial baseplates under physiological loading conditions. J Arthroplasty 2012;27(4):648–54.

39. Lewis PL, Rorabeck CH, Bourne RB. Screw osteolysis after cementless total knee replacement. Clin Orthop Relat Res 1995;321:173–7.

40. Bhimji S, Meneghini RM. Micromotion of cementless tibial baseplates: keels with adjuvant pegs offer more stability than pegs alone. J Arthroplasty 2014;29(7):1503–6.

41. Dumbleton J, Manley MT. Hydroxyapatite-coated prostheses in total hip and knee arthroplasty. J Bone Joint Surg Am 2004;86(11):2526–40.

42. Avila JD, Stenberg K, Bose S, et al. Hydroxyapatite reinforced Ti6Al4V composites for load-bearing implants. Acta Biomater 2021;123:379–92.

43. Dalton JE, Cook SD, Thomas KA, et al. The effect of operative fit and hydroxyapatite coating on the mechanical and biological response to porous implants. J Bone Joint Surg Am 1995;77(1):97–110.

44. Bellemans J. Osseointegration in porous coated knee arthroplasty. The influence of component coating type in sheep. Acta Orthop Scand Suppl 1999;288:1–35.

45. Li G, Wang L, Pan W, et al. In vitro and in vivo study of additive manufactured porous Ti6Al4V scaffolds for repairing bone defects. Sci Rep 2016;6:34072.

46. Karageorgiou V, Kaplan D. Porosity of 3D biomaterial scaffolds and osteogenesis. Biomaterials 2005;26(27):5474–91.

47. Khosla S, Westendorf JJ, Mödder UI. Concise review: Insights from normal bone remodeling and stem cell-based therapies for bone repair. Stem Cell 2010;28(12):2124–8.

48. Ng J, Spiller K, Bernhard J, et al. Biomimetic Approaches for Bone Tissue Engineering. Tissue Eng Part B Rev 2017;23(5):480–93.

49. Ortiz-Hernandez M, Rappe KS, Molmeneu M, et al. Two Different Strategies to Enhance Osseointegration in Porous Titanium: Inorganic Thermo-Chemical Treatment Versus Organic Coating by Peptide Adsorption. Int J Mol Sci 2018;19(9):2574.

50. Rappe KS, Ortiz-Hernandez M, Punset M, et al. On-Growth and In-Growth Osseointegration Enhancement in PM Porous Ti-Scaffolds by Two Different Bioactivation Strategies: Alkali Thermochemical Treatment and RGD Peptide Coating. Int J Mol Sci 2022;23(3):1750.

51. Turner TM, Urban RM, Sumner DR, et al. Bone ingrowth into the tibial component of a canine total condylar knee replacement prosthesis. J Orthop Res 1989;7(6):893–901.

52. Nilsson KG, Kärrholm J, Carlsson L, et al. Hydroxyapatite coating versus cemented fixation of the tibial component in total knee arthroplasty: Prospective randomized comparison of hydroxyapatite-coated and cemented tibial components with 5-year follow-up using radiostereometry. J Arthroplasty 1999;14(1):9–20.

53. Carlsson Å, Björkman A, Besjakov J, et al. Cemented tibial component fixation performs better than cementless fixation. Acta Orthop 2005;76(3):362–9.

54. Hansson U, Ryd L, Toksvig-Larsen S. A randomised RSA study of Peri-Apatite™ HA coating of a total knee prosthesis. Knee 2008;15(3):211–6.

55. Henricson A, Linder L, Nilsson KG. A trabecular metal tibial component in total knee replacement in patients younger than 60 years: A TWO-YEAR RADIOSTEREOPHOTOGRAMMETRIC ANALYSIS. The Journal of Bone & Joint Surgery British Volume 2008;90-B(12):1585–93.

56. Stilling M, Madsen F, Odgaard A, et al. Superior fixation of pegged trabecular metal over screw-fixed pegged porous titanium fiber mesh. Acta Orthop 2011;82(2):177–86.

57. Ryd L, Albrektsson BE, Carlsson L, et al. Roentgen stereophotogrammetric analysis as a predictor of mechanical loosening of knee prostheses. The Journal of Bone & Joint Surgery British Volume 1995;77-B(3):377–83.

58. Pijls BG, Valstar ER, Nouta KA, et al. Early migration of tibial components is associated with late revision. Acta Orthopaedica 2012;614–24.

59. Andersen MR, Winther NS, Lind T, et al. Low Preoperative BMD Is Related to High Migration of Tibia Components in Uncemented TKA—92 Patients in a Combined DEXA and RSA Study With 2-Year Follow-Up. J Arthroplasty 2017;32(7):2141–6.

60. Petersen MM, Nielsen PT, Lebech A, et al. Preoperative bone mineral density of the proximal tibia and migration of the tibial component after uncemented total knee arthroplasty. J Arthroplasty 1999;14(1):77–81.

61. Lee RW, Volz RG, Sheridan DC. The Role of Fixation and Bone Quality on the Mechanical Stability of Tibial Knee Components. Clin Orthop Relat Res 1991;273:177.

62. Tu KN, Lie JD, Wan CKV, et al. Osteoporosis: A Review of Treatment Options. P T 2018;43(2):92–104.

63. Chesnut CH III, Skag A, Christiansen C, et al. Effects of Oral Ibandronate Administered Daily or Intermittently on Fracture Risk in Postmenopausal Osteoporosis. J Bone Miner Res 2004;19(8):1241–9.

64. Harris ST, Watts NB, Genant HK, et al. Effects of Risedronate Treatment on Vertebral and Nonvertebral Fractures in Women With Postmenopausal OsteoporosisA Randomized Controlled Trial. JAMA 1999;282(14):1344–52.

65. Reginster JY, Minne HW, Sorensen OH, et al. Randomized Trial of the Effects of Risedronate on Vertebral Fractures in Women with Established Postmenopausal Osteoporosis. Osteoporos Int 2000;11(1):83–91.

66. Black DM, Delmas PD, Eastell R, et al. Once-Yearly Zoledronic Acid for Treatment of Post-menopausal Osteoporosis. N Engl J Med 2007; 356(18):1809–22.

67. Cummings SR, Black DM, Thompson DE, et al. Effect of Alendronate on Risk of Fracture in Women With Low Bone Density but Without Vertebral FracturesResults From the Fracture Intervention Trial. JAMA 1998;280(24):2077–82.

68. Mcclung MR, Wasnich RD, Recker R, et al. Oral Daily Ibandronate Prevents Bone Loss in Early Postmenopausal Women Without Osteoporosis. J Bone Miner Res 2004;19(1):11–8.

69. Seeman E, Delmas PD. Bone Quality — The Material and Structural Basis of Bone Strength and Fragility. N Engl J Med 2006;354(21):2250–61.

70. Osterhoff G, Morgan EF, Shefelbine SJ, et al. Bone mechanical properties and changes with osteoporosis. Injury 2016;47(Suppl 2):S11–20.

71. Vall H, Parmar M. Teriparatide. In: StatPearls. StatPearls Publishing; 2023. Available at: http://www.ncbi.nlm.nih.gov/books/NBK559248/. [Accessed 23 October 2023].

72. Canalis E. MANAGEMENT OF ENDOCRINE DISEASE: Novel anabolic treatments for osteoporosis. Eur J Endocrinol 2018;178(2):R33–44.

73. Jilka RL. Molecular and cellular mechanisms of the anabolic effect of intermittent PTH. Bone 2007; 40(6):1434–46.

74. Lee M, Partridge NC. Parathyroid hormone signaling in bone and kidney. Curr Opin Nephrol Hypertens 2009;18(4):298–302.

75. van Loon CJ, Oyen WJ, de Waal Malefijt MC, et al. Distal femoral bone mineral density after total knee arthroplasty: a comparison with general bone mineral density. Arch Orthop Trauma Surg 2001;121(5):282–5.

76. Winther N, Jensen C, Petersen M, et al. Changes in bone mineral density of the proximal tibia after uncemented total knee arthroplasty. A prospective randomized study. Int Orthop 2016;40(2):285–94.

77. Huang CC, Jiang CC, Hsieh CH, et al. Local bone quality affects the outcome of prosthetic total knee arthroplasty. J Orthop Res 2016;34(2):240–8.

78. Petersen MM, Lauritzen JB, Pedersen JG, et al. Decreased bone density of the distal femur after uncemented knee arthroplasty. A 1-year follow-up of 29 knees. Acta Orthop Scand 1996;67(4):339–44.

79. Lin T, Yan SG, Cai XZ, et al. Bisphosphonates for periprosthetic bone loss after joint arthroplasty: a meta-analysis of 14 randomized controlled trials. Osteoporos Int 2012;23(6):1823–34.

80. Khatod M, Inacio MCS, Dell RM, et al. Association of Bisphosphonate Use and Risk of Revision After THA: Outcomes From a US Total Joint Replacement Registry. Clin Orthop Relat Res 2015; 473(11):3412–20.

81. Ro DH, Jin H, Park JY, et al. The use of bisphosphonates after joint arthroplasty is associated with lower implant revision rate. Knee Surg Sports Traumatol Arthrosc 2019;27(7):2082–9.

82. Namba RS, Inacio MCS, Cheetham TC, et al. Lower Total Knee Arthroplasty Revision Risk Associated With Bisphosphonate Use, Even in Patients With Normal Bone Density. J Arthroplasty 2016;31(2):537–41.

83. Prieto-Alhambra D, Lalmohamed A, Abrahamsen B, et al. Oral bisphosphonate use and total knee/hip implant survival: validation of results in an external population-based cohort. Arthritis Rheumatol 2014;66(11):3233–40.

84. Dell RM, Adams AL, Greene DF, et al. Incidence of atypical nontraumatic diaphyseal fractures of the femur. J Bone Miner Res 2012;27(12):2544–50.

85. Nam D, Lawrie CM, Salih R, et al. Cemented Versus Cementless Total Knee Arthroplasty of the Same Modern Design: A Prospective, Randomized Trial. J Bone Joint Surg Am 2019; 101(13):1185–92.

86. Liu Y, Zeng Y, Wu Y, et al. A comprehensive comparison between cementless and cemented fixation in the total knee arthroplasty: an updated systematic review and meta-analysis. J Orthop Surg Res 2021;16(1):176.

87. Chen C, Li R. Cementless versus cemented total knee arthroplasty in young patients: a meta-analysis of randomized controlled trials. J Orthop Surg Res 2019;14(1):262.

88. Mont MA, Pivec R, Issa K, et al. Long-term implant survivorship of cementless total knee arthroplasty: a systematic review of the literature and meta-analysis. J Knee Surg 2014;27(5):369–76.

89. Therbo M, Petersen MM, Varmarken JE, et al. Influence of pre-operative bone mineral content of the proximal tibia on revision rate after uncemented knee arthroplasty. J Bone Joint Surg Br 2003;85(7):975–9.

90. Dixon P, Parish EN, Chan B, et al. Hydroxyapatite-coated, cementless total knee replacement in patients aged 75 years and over. The Journal of Bone & Joint Surgery British 2004;86-B(2): 200–4.

91. Gibbons JP, Cassidy RS, Bryce L, et al. Is Cementless Total Knee Arthroplasty Safe in Women Over 75 Y of Age? J Arthroplasty 2023;38(4):691–9.

92. Goh GS, Fillingham YA, Ong CB, et al. Redefining Indications for Modern Cementless Total Knee Arthroplasty: Clinical Outcomes and Survivorship in Patients >75 Years Old. J Arthroplasty 2022; 37(3):476–81.e1.

93. American Joint Replacement Registry (AJRR). 2022 Annual report. Rosemont, IL: American Academy of Orthopaedic Surgeons (AAOS); 2022. Available at: https://connect.registryapps.net/hubfs/PDFs%20and%20PPTs/2022%20AJRR%

20Annual%20Report.pdf?utm_referrer=https%3A%2F%2Fconnect.registryapps.net%2F.

94. Lewis PL, W-Dahl A, Robertsson O, et al. The effect of patient and prosthesis factors on revision rates after total knee replacement using a multi-registry meta-analytic approach. Acta Orthop 2022;93:284–93.

95. Witmer DK, Meneghini RM. Cementless total knee arthroplasty: Patient selection and surgical techniques to optimize outcomes. Semin Arthroplasty 2018;29(1):50–4.

96. Kamath AF, Siddiqi A, Malkani AL, et al. Cementless Fixation in Primary Total Knee Arthroplasty: Historical Perspective to Contemporary Application. JAAOS - Journal of the American Academy of Orthopaedic Surgeons 2021;29(8):e363.

97. King BA, Malkani AL. Cementless Total Knee Arthroplasty. In: Hansen E, Kühn KD, editors. Essentials of cemented knee arthroplasty. Springer;

2022. p. 365–76. https://doi.org/10.1007/978-3-662-63113-3_32.

98. Berend ME, Small SR, Ritter MA, et al. The Effects of Bone Resection Depth and Malalignment on Strain in the Proximal Tibia After Total Knee Arthroplasty. J Arthroplasty 2010;25(2):314–8.

99. Andersen MR, Winther N, Lind T, et al. Tibial Component Undersizing Is Related to High Degrees of Implant Migration Following Cementless Total Knee Arthroplasty. JB JS Open Access 2023; 8(3). e23.00032.

100. Dalury DF. Cementless total knee arthroplasty: current concepts review. Bone Joint Lett J 2016; 98-B(7):867–73.

101. Laforest G, Kostretzis L, Kiss MO, et al. Restricted kinematic alignment leads to uncompromised osseointegration of cementless total knee arthroplasty. Knee Surg Sports Traumatol Arthrosc 2022; 30(2):705–12.

Pediatrics

Perioperative Evaluation and Management of Children with Osteoporosis and Low Bone Mineral Density

Jordan D. Ross, MD[a],*, Alicia Diaz-Thomas, MD, MPH[b,c]

KEYWORDS

- Perioperative • Bisphosphonate • Osteoporosis • Osteogenesis imperfecta • Osteotomy
- Pediatric • Bone heath optimization

KEY POINTS

- The diagnosis of osteoporosis in children is based on both bone density measurements and fracture history.
- For children undergoing surgery for fracture, preoperative suspicion for osteoporosis based on fracture history and exposures can facilitate multidisciplinary evaluation and initiation of bisphosphonate therapy when indicated.
- Recent evidence does not support routinely holding bisphosphonates after osteotomy, but discussion as part of perioperative bone health optimization is warranted.
- Atypical femur fractures and osteonecrosis of the jaw are reported as bony adverse effects in adults treated with bisphosphonates but seem less common in children.

INTRODUCTION

As medical and surgical treatment options for patients with osteoporosis improve, management strategies have become more robust but also more complex. Multidisciplinary teams including orthopedists, endocrinologists, and physical therapists are needed to develop coordinated treatment plans to offer their patients. This collaborative approach is important for perioperative planning, as well.

Most often, pediatric patients who are managed by multidisciplinary bone teams have underlying insults to bone, which are often classified as either osteoporosis or low bone mass. Osteoporosis in pediatrics typically refers to a specific clinical scenario, whereas low bone mass reflects a low Z-score (Z < −2 standard deviations) on dual-energy X-ray absorptiometry (DXA) of various measurements, ideally matched by age and height. Osteopenia is typically a term not used in pediatrics but often used in adults to denote a particular T-score on DXA.

In terms of bone mineral density (BMD) evaluation for children, DXA of the lumbar spine and total body less head are standard measurements. However, in patients for whom positioning, hardware, or other factors hinder accurate readings, other sites are used, including the forearm and lateral distal femur.[1] It is important to measure the same sites (ideally obtained from the same machine) for consistent comparison over time. Some sites may accrue orthopedic hardware throughout the person's life, affecting BMD measurements. In addition, BMD measurements on DXA depend on the reference database applied.[2]

---

[a] University of Tennessee Health Science Center, Faculty Office Building, Room 119, 49 North Dunlap, Memphis, TN 38103, USA; [b] Division of Pediatric Endocrinology, University of Tennessee Heath Science Center, Suite 1006, 910 Madison Avenue, Memphis, TN 38163, USA; [c] Division of Pediatric Endocrinology, Le Bonheur Children's Hospital, Memphis, TN, USA
* Corresponding author. Faculty Office Building, Room 119, 49 North Dunlap, Memphis, TN 38103.
E-mail address: jross27@uthsc.edu

Orthop Clin N Am 55 (2024) 345–353
https://doi.org/10.1016/j.ocl.2023.11.003
0030-5898/24/

The pediatric position statement from the International Society for Clinical Densitometry (ISCD) provides a helpful framework for a working definition of osteoporosis in children.[3] Typically, at least 1 of the following clinical scenarios is met:

- At least 1 vertebral compression fracture not associated with localized disease or high-impact trauma
- A BMD Z-score ≤ -2.0 standard deviation and a "clinically significant fracture history"
  1. At least 2 long-bone fractures by age 10 or
  2. At least 3 long-bone fractures at any age up to 19 years of age

Despite this important guidance from the ISCD and other organizations, the definition of pediatric osteoporosis is still debated. Determining the threshold at which the mechanism of injury for a fracture is low impact (denoting fragility) is not entirely clear. Furthermore, bone mass may be recovered over time in a growing child, particularly if exacerbating factors like chronic glucocorticoids[4] or delayed puberty are withdrawn. Vertebral fractures may undergo reshaping,[2] even without pharmacologic therapy; this phenomenon seems particularly common in children with secondary osteoporosis.[5] Due to these uncertainties and caveats, the diagnosis of osteoporosis in any child must be applied thoughtfully to avoid inappropriate treatment.

Often, treatment of osteoporosis includes consideration of pharmaceutical agents, adjustment of high-risk medications, and lifestyle changes (nutrition, mobility). Bisphosphonates are a standard of care for adults with osteoporosis and used "off-label" (despite having decades' worth of data) in children with osteoporosis.[6] The timing of these medications in the perioperative setting is an area of active research; there are no clear standards in terms of how long to withhold bisphosphonates prior to significant orthopedic surgery, nor how long to wait before restarting them after surgery. Other classes of drugs used in adult populations for their osteoanabolic effects have even more limited data in children but are discussed briefly, as well. This review discusses various approaches to pharmacology and other considerations in the perioperative management of children with osteoporosis.

PATIENT EVALUATION OVERVIEW IN THE PERIOPERATIVE PERIOD

Bone health optimization (BHO) is an emerging strategy for improving postoperative outcomes in older adults undergoing significant orthopedic surgery.[7] Pertinent elements applicable to children with osteoporosis include biochemical evaluation for derangements in bone metabolism, for example, changes in serum levels of calcium, phosphorus, magnesium, parathyroid hormone, and 25-hydroxyvitamin D, as well as preoperative evaluation for appropriateness of bisphosphonate therapy. There is no consensus statement recommending routine laboratory tests, but many patients who have been evaluated by an endocrinologist, particularly those on bisphosphonate therapy, may have these laboratory values monitored periodically.

Adequate vitamin D status may optimize skeletal response to bisphosphonates (though this is less studied in children).[8] Conclusions on the benefit of vitamin D supplementation on perioperative orthopedic outcomes are ongoing,[9] but this has not been well studied in children with osteoporosis. It is also not clear what role vitamin D deficiency has in outcomes of children undergoing orthopedic surgery.[10] Without adequate vitamin D stores, patients treated with bisphosphonates may be at higher risk of hypocalcemia.[11]

During preoperative consultations for orthopedic surgery, a thorough history is indicated to assess nutrition and mobility status prior to surgery. Pediatric malnutrition, which can generally be considered as a net deficit of nutrients that impacts growth and development, is associated with a higher risk of postoperative complications in children who undergo surgical management of scoliosis.[12,13] When available, evaluation by a dietitian can be particularly helpful for assessing a child's dietary habits and nutritional status. Importantly, malnutrition and immobility both contribute to secondary osteoporosis in children.[14] Thus, it is important that nutritional status be normalized prior to any scheduled orthopedic intervention.

The role of preoperative DXA is unclear when scheduling elective surgeries in patients with low BMD, particularly with regard to timing and patient population, given that the diagnosis and treatment of pediatric osteoporosis is not solely dependent on DXA parameters. A multi-center research team in the United States retrospectively assessed the preoperative management of children who had low BMD-related terminology in their medical records prior to spinal fusion. A significantly higher proportion of patients who had preoperative DXA received bisphosphonate therapy (81% vs 52%, $P = .03$); however, the authors acknowledged that the absence of clinical guidelines impacted standardization of care.[15] The patients who were classified as having osteoporosis had a more complicated postoperative course. This research group noted more research is needed to understand whether preoperative DXA, and in some cases, intervention with intravenous bisphosphonates, in medically complicated children is a better predictor of outcome after spinal fusion than the patients' clinical diagnoses alone.

A recent neurosurgical guideline resulting from a systematic review concerning preoperative evaluation of adult patients undergoing spinal surgery recommends assessments of bone density by DXA and computed tomography (CT) scan as well as measurement and treatment of vitamin D insufficiency. The authors noted that while perioperative treatment with teriparatide seemed to improve outcomes, data were less clear for bisphosphonate treatment.[16] Similarly, for elective orthopedic surgeries in children with a clinical context concerning for osteoporosis (Box 1),[17] the biochemical evaluation (serum levels of calcium, phosphorus, magnesium, parathyroid hormone, and 25-hydroxyvitamin D) is indicated and a preoperative DXA with vertebral fracture assessment may be helpful. Discussion with an endocrinologist to determine optimal sites of measurement is important, again considering potential implantation of hardware. The pediatric position paper from the ISCD is also a helpful reference.[3] There is a degree of bias, as outcomes of patients who receive a preoperative DXA (ie, carry a certain degree of risk for low BMD) may be confounded by any previous pharmacotherapy as a response to the DXA.[15]

Because bisphosphonates can promote stronger bones prior to surgery, a rigorous evaluation for osteoporosis and initiation of bisphosphonate therapy can provide an optimal perioperative environment for these patients. Box 2 highlights various medications[18] and other exposures that increase the risk for low BMD and may indicate the need for evaluation, including endocrinology referral, prior to elective surgery.

Although BMD is the direct data point derived from DXA scan, BMD may not correlate directly with bone strength; for example, a

Box 1
Clinical features that raise suspicion for osteoporosis in children
History of vertebral fracture[2]
History of multiple long-bone fractures[2]
Family history of significant fractures[17]

Box 2
Exposures that increase risk for low bone mineral density
Chronic glucocorticoids more than 3 months[4]
Antiepileptic drugs[18]
Long-term limited mobility for age[14]
Delayed puberty[14]

growing skeleton may be stronger over time even as BMD measurements are lower due to increasing bone size.[19] While radial BMD measurements on DXA trended with measures of radial bone strength on peripheral quantitative CT in adolescent females,[20] this association has not been established for all sites of measurement within the skeleton, nor for all pediatric populations. Similarly, gains in BMD associated with bisphosphonate therapy may not equate with gains in bone strength.[21]

Perioperative Strategies for Incident Fractures

While multidisciplinary planning for elective orthopedic surgery can be stepwise and iterative, some children with osteoporosis present with an incident fracture that needs urgent intervention. In these cases, the workup may be performed in parallel with treatment. Postoperative multidisciplinary collaboration is warranted, again with the goal of promoting BHO.

It is appropriate to check 25-hydroxyvitamin D and calcium levels for a patient presenting with an incident fracture requiring urgent surgical intervention, particularly if no recent baseline is available.[22] There are limited data that vitamin D supplementation improves outcomes in this situation, but obtaining a blood level permits treatment of vitamin D deficiency for prospective bone health. Hypocalcemia often warrants emergent treatment and a multidisciplinary approach, including electrocardiogram (EKG) to assess for changes in the QT interval. Children with QT changes (or those who may experience seizure as a result of hypocalcemia) should have intravenous calcium gluconate provided, as well as oral calcium, until the EKG changes resolve. The oral calcium supplementation is typically continued for months. While a parathyroid hormone level is critical for biochemical information about metabolic bone health, the level may be elevated in the setting of acute fracture[23] and can be repeated after several months of bone healing.

In terms of bisphosphonate treatment in the setting of acute fracture, its role in bone healing (whether operative or not) has limited data, and more research is needed in this area. This approach is not currently standard practice.

PHARMACOLOGY TREATMENT OPTIONS: PEDIATRIC USE OF BISPHOSPHONATES
Osteogenesis Imperfecta
Much of the evidence for pediatric bisphosphonate use arises from their application to children with osteogenesis imperfecta (OI). It is important to continue bisphosphonates throughout growing time to limit pain and fracture rates for these children.[24] For patients with OI, improvement in BMD and fracture risk after bisphosphonate therapy are variable and have been associated with the specific phenotype.[25] Due to the effect of decreasing bone turnover, previous bisphosphonate therapy is evidenced on radiographs as sclerotic lines in the metaphyses of growing bones in patients with OI.[24] As these children continue to have long-bone fractures, straightening may be required with intramedullary rodding.[26]

Previously, Munns and colleagues[27] investigated outcomes in children with OI treated with pamidronate. On multivariate analysis, pamidronate use was not associated with delayed healing after fracture but was associated with delayed healing after osteotomy (osteotomy line visible at 12 months after the surgery). However, the number of weeks since the last pamidronate infusion and before the next pamidronate infusion were not associated with the risk of delayed healing after osteotomy. These results prompted the Shriners Hospital for Children to modify their protocol by withholding bisphosphonate for 4 months after osteotomy.[26] This group reported a lower incidence of delayed osteotomy healing after practice changes to osteotome (vs oscillating power saw) for surgical approach and zoledronic acid (vs pamidronate) for their standard bisphosphonate.[26]

A report on osteotomies and Fassier-Duval nailing by Azzam and colleagues[28] included children with OI who had been receiving cyclic pamidronate therapy. There was no adjustment by the medical team to the bisphosphonate treatment cycle relative to the surgical procedure in this midterm report and the investigators did not report that the surgeries were scheduled at particular intervals relative to the infusion. Azzam and colleagues[28] did not note any increase in nonunion or delayed healing despite not adjusting the bisphosphonate cycle. The investigators acknowledge that the lack of evidence relative to bisphosphonate treatment

and orthopedic surgery timing has led to a variability in strategies for perioperative bisphosphonate. They do not go as far as to use their experience as evidence of a lack of adverse effects but note that there is a "consensus" regarding the generally beneficial effect of bisphosphonate therapy on orthopedic procedural results.[28]

A research group at the University of Colorado in the United States performed a retrospective review of patients younger than 19 years of age with at least 1 Fassier-Duval rod implantation in the context of OI. Treatment with bisphosphonates was captured as a variable, but in this small population (n = 13), a statistical association with bisphosphonate therapy and time to rod failure was not available.[29] A larger study with specifics on bisphosphonate use (timing of doses before and after rod implantation, and so forth) may provide more insight into the benefit of this drug class for optimal outcomes after rod implantation.

A study out of Cairo University in Egypt looked at the effects of pamidronate (administered via the Glorieux protocol) in addition to surgical correction for patients with OI. The investigators discussed the reported benefits of bisphosphonates in this population, as well as unanswered questions related to dosage and duration.[30] There were 2 groups of patients: group 1 was identified as a retrospective group who had received surgical correction of femur, tibia, or humerus fracture (intramedullary pinning with plaster fixation) at 1 hospital and group 2 was a prospective group at another institution who received the same surgical techniques for the same areas and were treated with pamidronate infusions starting 3 weeks postoperatively and continuing for a period ranging from 8 months to 2 years and 8 months. The group of patients who received pamidronate after surgery had improved bone mass and mobility-related outcomes than the patients treated with surgery alone. Although the 2 study groups in this project were managed at different hospitals by the same surgeons, there are limited comparisons between the 2 intervention groups. A future trial with randomization to either bisphosphonate or placebo may assess effects on perioperative outcomes with fewer confounding variables.

Other
In pediatric patients with osteotomy, distraction osteogenesis (DO) may be used to correct deformity while lengthening a bone after osteotomy.[31] While it is not standard practice,

bisphosphonate therapy has been used for anabolic effect in patients undergoing DO after osteotomy for limb lengthening.[32] In the Kiely study, research participants received a bisphosphonate infusion an average of 170 days (range 124–252 days) after fixation with an Ilizarov external fixator, after a clinical assessment of inadequate and stalled postoperative growth. In other words, there was a perioperative period of monitoring bone growth prior to intervening with bisphosphonate therapy. This may be another technique for applying bisphosphonates after osteotomy in patients who are most likely to benefit or most likely to have additional complications without this therapy. More research on the benefits of this application of bisphosphonates is needed, as this class's antiresorptive effects may not directly translate into net increase in bone formation.

Bisphosphonate Dosing

The dosing of bisphosphonates varies depending on the indication and other patient factors. For young children, including those with OI, zoledronic acid is often given as 0.025 mg/kg every 3 months; the doses can be increased and given less often in older children (0.05 mg/kg every 6 months).[6] Pamidronate is another commonly used option with a more complex dosing schedule, including a daily infusion for 3 days as a single course.[6]

Because of the off-label use of bisphosphonates in children with OI and other forms of osteoporosis, the dosing schedule can be adjusted to fit the clinical context. Some patients find that their bony pain is better controlled with more frequent infusions at lower doses, and this shared decision-making with patients and their families allows for more family-focused care. The first bisphosphonate infusion can also be given at a lower dose (eg, 0.0125 mg/kg for an infant with OI) to assess a patient's response. A zoledronic acid infusion can typically be administered within a 2-hour time period, and a slower infusion rate can be applied for children who have experienced a more severe infusion-related rash or other inflammatory reaction (**Box 3**). More recently, several groups have been investigating lower doses of bisphosphonates, particularly for children who are receiving these for longer periods of time.[33,34]

TREATMENT COMPLICATIONS: ADVERSE EFFECTS OF BISPHOSPHONATES

While **Box 3** provides a more complete list of adverse effects of bisphosphonates,[11] including

Box 3
Adverse effects of bisphosphonates
Acute inflammatory reaction[35]
Hypocalcemia[11]
Hypophosphatemia[11]
Osteonecrosis of the jaw
Atypical femur fracture

an acute inflammatory reaction,[35] bony complications are described in more detail in the following paragraphs. The acute inflammatory reaction is common within the first few hours to days after a bisphosphonate infusion and can include fever, myalgias, headache, and other flulike symptoms. Acetaminophen can be given for the 3 days after the infusion to prevent or mitigate these symptoms, and premedicating with acetaminophen on the day of the infusion is also appropriate.[35]

Atypical femur fracture (AFF) and osteonecrosis of the jaw (ONJ) have been associated with bisphosphonate use. Despite some evidence supporting this association, there are debates within the metabolic bone community and limited pediatric data. Black and colleagues[36] reviewed fracture data from 3 bisphosphonate trials comprising more than 14,000 women and defined atypia as particular features (eg, oblique or transverse fracture) for fractures in certain locations (below the lesser trochanter and above the distal metaphyseal flare, ie, subtrochanteric and diaphyseal fractures). Ultimately, bisphosphonate use did not seem to confer additional risk of AFF, though the studies were underpowered to detect a difference. Black and colleagues[37] followed this work with a study of more than 196,000 women treated with bisphosphonates and cited 277 AFF, with higher risk associated with longer duration of bisphosphonate use.

The data on AFF are more limited in pediatric practice. Notably, a cohort of 123 patients followed at Cincinnati Children's Hospital Medical Center had no reports of either AFF or ONJ after an average of 3.8 years of follow-up (468 patient years of bisphosphonate exposure).[11] With evidence again coming from the OI community, Trejo and colleagues[38] reviewed the femur fractures of 119 children with OI; for the 36 fractures occurring in nondeformed femurs, AFF risk was not associated with history of bisphosphonate use on linear regression analysis. The investigators noted the retrospective nature of their study.

Data on the risk and incidence of ONJ in children treated with bisphosphonates are also limited. For a group of 42 children with osteoporosis (35 of whom had OI) treated with bisphosphonates out of Australia, all underwent dental assessment with no evidence of ONJ; average duration of treatment with pamidronate or zoledronic acid was 6.5 years.[39] A review summarized the findings of 10 studies reporting bisphosphonate use in 572 patients with OI (age 0.2–23.4 years) with no reports of ONJ.[40] The investigators noted the heterogeneity of bisphosphonate protocols and need for longitudinal studies to provide clearer guidelines; it is not known why ONJ seems less common in this population.[40] A more recent retrospective study of 122 children treated with antiresorptive therapy (all but 3 patients received a bisphosphonate) cited no cases of ONJ after an average of 4.89 years of follow-up.[41]

FUTURE DIRECTIONS: REVIEW OF ADULT DATA

The more extensive experience with bisphosphonates in adults provides other opportunities for applications to pediatric orthopedic care. Lozano-Calderon and colleagues[42] published a review of bisphosphonate use in the context of orthopedics in 2014. While pediatric use is considered (including the acknowledgment of limited evidence at the time), bisphosphonate use in adults is discussed. Perioperative management of patients on bisphosphonates is not a primary focus of Lozano-Calderon's[42] article, but several pertinent indications are addressed.

There may be a role in bisphosphonate use to encourage bony union after surgery. In adults, bisphosphonates have been used for healing after osteotomy in patients without osteoporosis. In a cohort of 46 adult patients undergoing high tibial osteotomy for osteoarthritis, randomization to 4 mg of zoledronic acid (vs placebo) was associated with increased extraction torque force, a measure of fixation, in patients treated with a standard pin.[43] For a group of patients with osteoporosis who underwent anterior cervical discectomy and fusion, randomization to 5 mg of zoledronic acid at 5 days after surgery was associated with a higher stability of spine fusion, assessed as grade 1 or 2 osteogenesis. 76.2% of patients in the intervention arm versus 45.5% of patients in the control arm had achieved this level of osteogenesis at 3 months; and 90.5% and 68.2%, respectively, at 6 months. The group treated with zoledronic also had significantly lower markers of bone turnover, procollagen type 1 N-propeptide and C-terminal telopeptide of type 1 collagen.[44]

Other pharmacologic agents with antiresorptive properties have been studied in adults with metabolic bone disorders. Cheng and colleagues[45] reviewed the use of combination teriparatide and denosumab with favorable outcomes after spinal fusion, defined as higher fusion rate. Denosumab is a monoclonal antibody against RANKL (receptor activator of nuclear factor kappa B ligand), and its effect is to inhibit osteoclast activation and thus bone degradation.[46] Off-label use of denosumab is reported in children with OI[46] and other metabolic bone conditions, but more research is needed to study its perioperative benefit in both adults and children, particularly as monotherapy. There are several other medications, including sclerostin inhibitors, that are undergoing clinical trials for use in patients with OI and may provide yet another tool for perioperative management.

The Santa Fe Bone Symposium reviewed preoperative bone health assessment, similar to the BHO concept discussed earlier. The authors focused on spinal fusion specifically and noted that no guidelines exist. DXA and evaluation for spine fractures can be considered in older populations and those with other risk factors, including chronic glucocorticoid use.[47] As noted in **Box 2**, it is important to consider a person's bone health prior to elective orthopedic surgery. Underlying osteoporosis can be evaluated and managed perioperatively for optimal outcomes. While the etiologies of osteoporosis in children differ from adult-onset osteoporosis (and the underlying physiology of bone accrual is different, as well), the general principles are helpful.

Mugge and colleagues[48] investigated the association between osteoporosis and outcomes after thoracolumbar fusion in adults. The patients with osteoporosis had a higher incidence of instrumentation failure. The conclusion was the importance of preoperative evaluation for osteoporosis by a multidisciplinary team with initiation of pharmacologic therapy before surgery if indicated.

Formal guidelines for perioperative bisphosphonate use and for the interface between orthopedic and metabolic bone health are limited. Nonetheless, the vast number of studies in adults, including implementation of newer surgical techniques and pharmacologic therapies, is an important resource that can carefully be considered and incorporated into pediatric care, as well.

SUMMARY

The diagnosis of osteoporosis in children is complex and requires longitudinal data on BMD in the context of fracture history. A low threshold of suspicion based on clinical features and risk factors for osteoporosis can allow for an appropriate evaluation by a multidisciplinary team so that BHO can be targeted for each patient.

In children with osteoporosis, bisphosphonate therapy is a well-studied and standard treatment. While there has been a historical concern for impaired healing after osteotomy in patients with bisphosphonate exposure, more recent data suggest this concern may not be as great with current bisphosphonate protocols and surgical approaches. It may not be necessary to adjust or hold bisphosphonate therapy, and in fact there may be benefits on postoperative recovery of the bone. Much of the available data come from populations with OI, but similar investigations are being conducted in other populations with orthopedic and metabolic bone-related conditions.

It is important to consider the side effects of bisphosphonates and adjust the dosing strategy for each patient accordingly. While ONJ and AFF are the side effects particularly noteworthy for the orthopedic surgeon, the association of these conditions with bisphosphonates is weaker in children than in adults for incompletely understood reasons. Again, further study is needed to quantify the risk more accurately and to understand why the phenomena seem more commonly reported in adults than in children.

Bisphosphonates are the typical pharmacologic arm of a more comprehensive strategy for optimal bone health that includes physical therapy and mobility, a diet rich in calcium and phosphorus, and vitamin D optimization. These tools should be considered and employed by a multidisciplinary team and applied to each patient and his/her particular surgical needs.

CLINICS CARE POINTS

- Use both BMD measurements (compared to appropriate reference ranges) and fracture history to arrive at a diagnosis of osteoporosis in children.
- BHO allows orthopedic surgeons, endocrinologists, and other team members to formulate a perioperative plan that considers bisphosphonates and other nonsurgical options to supplement surgical outcomes.
- It remains uncertain, but recent evidence suggests that bisphosphonates may not interfere with healing after osteotomy; at the same time, the benefits of this drug class for perioperative outcomes require more study.

- ONJ and AFFs are bisphosphonate-associated adverse events but may be less common in children than in adults, though longer follow-up may be needed for a more complete picture.

DISCLOSURE

There are no commercial or financial conflicts of interest for either author. There are no funding sources.

REFERENCES

1. Weber DR, Boyce A, Gordon C, et al. The Utility of DXA Assessment at the Forearm, Proximal Femur, and Lateral Distal Femur, and Vertebral Fracture Assessment in the Pediatric Population: 2019 ISCD Official Position. J Clin Densitom 2019;22(4):567–89.
2. Ward LM, Weber DR, Munns CF, et al. A Contemporary View of the Definition and Diagnosis of Osteoporosis in Children and Adolescents. J Clin Endocrinol Metab 2020;105(5):e2088–97.
3. Pediatric Positions. The International Society for Clinical Densitometry. Accessed October 21, 2023, 2023. https://iscd.org/learn/official-positions/pediatric-positions/.
4. Ward LM. Glucocorticoid-Induced Osteoporosis: Why Kids Are Different. Front Endocrinol 2020;11:576.
5. Montero-Lopez R, Laurer E, Tischlinger K, et al. Spontaneous reshaping of vertebral fractures in an adolescent with osteogenesis imperfecta. Bone Rep 2022;16:101595.
6. Ciancia S, Hogler W, Sakkers RJB, et al. Osteoporosis in children and adolescents: how to treat and monitor? Eur J Pediatr 2023;182(2):501–11.
7. Kostenuik PJ, Binkley N, Anderson PA. Advances in Osteoporosis Therapy: Focus on Osteoanabolic Agents, Secondary Fracture Prevention, and Perioperative Bone Health. Curr Osteoporos Rep 2023. https://doi.org/10.1007/s11914-023-00793-8.
8. Mosali P, Bernard L, Wajed J, et al. Vitamin D status and parathyroid hormone concentrations influence the skeletal response to zoledronate and denosumab. Calcif Tissue Int 2014;94(5):553–9.
9. Morrison RJM, Fishley WG, Rankin KS, et al. The effect of vitamin D supplementation on outcomes following total hip or knee arthroplasty surgery: a rapid systematic review of current evidence. EFORT Open Rev 2022;7(5):305–11.
10. Parry J, Sullivan E, Scott AC. Vitamin D sufficiency screening in preoperative pediatric orthopaedic patients. J Pediatr Orthop 2011;31(3):331–3.
11. Nasomyont N, Hornung LN, Gordon CM, et al. Outcomes following intravenous bisphosphonate infusion in pediatric patients: A 7-year retrospective chart review. Bone 2019;121:60–7.

12. Becker P, Carney LN, Corkins MR, et al. Consensus statement of the Academy of Nutrition and Dietetics/American Society for Parenteral and Enteral Nutrition: indicators recommended for the identification and documentation of pediatric malnutrition (undernutrition). Nutr Clin Pract 2015;30(1):147–61.

13. Karls CA, Duey-Holtz A, Lampone OA, et al. Prevalence of malnutrition and its associated outcomes in pediatric patients with scoliosis undergoing elective posterior spinal fusion or spine growth modulation - a retrospective review. Stud Health Technol Inf 2021;280:235–40.

14. Bianchi ML. Causes of secondary pediatric osteoporosis. Pediatr Endocrinol Rev 2013;10(Suppl 2): 424–36.

15. Cohen LL, Berry JG, Ma NS, et al. Spinal Fusion in Pediatric Patients With Low Bone Density: Defining the Value of DXA. J Pediatr Orthop 2022;42(7): e713–9.

16. Dimar J, Bisson EF, Dhall S, et al. Congress of Neurological Surgeons Systematic Review and Evidence-Based Guidelines for Perioperative Spine: Preoperative Osteoporosis Assessment. Neurosurgery 2021;89(Suppl 1):S19–25.

17. Ciancia S, van Rijn RR, Hogler W, et al. Osteoporosis in children and adolescents: when to suspect and how to diagnose it. Eur J Pediatr 2022;181(7): 2549–61.

18. Miziak B, Blaszczyk B, Chroscinska-Krawczyk M, et al. The problem of osteoporosis in epileptic patients taking antiepileptic drugs. Expet Opin Drug Saf 2014;13(7):935–46.

19. Lindgren E, Rosengren BE, Karlsson MK. Does peak bone mass correlate with peak bone strength? Cross-sectional normative dual energy X-ray absorptiometry data in 1052 men aged 18-28 years. BMC Muscoskel Disord 2019;20(1):404.

20. Dowthwaite JN, Hickman RM, Kanaley JA, et al. Distal radius strength: a comparison of DXA-derived vs pQCT-measured parameters in adolescent females. J Clin Densitom 2009;12(1):42–53.

21. Szalay EA. Bisphosphonate use in children with pediatric osteoporosis and other bone conditions. J Pediatr Rehabil Med 2014;7(2):125–32.

22. Patterson JT, Tangtiphaiboontana J, Pandya NK. Management of Pediatric Femoral Neck Fracture. J Am Acad Orthop Surg 2018;26(12):411–9.

23. Karkenny AJ, Avarello J, Hanstein R, et al. Pediatric Fractures: Does Vitamin D Play a Role? J Pediatr Orthop 2023;43(8):492–7.

24. Robinson ME, Trejo P, Palomo T, et al. Osteogenesis Imperfecta: Skeletal Outcomes After Bisphosphonate Discontinuation at Final Height. J Bone Miner Res 2019;34(12):2198–204.

25. Sun L, Hu J, Liu J, et al. Relationship of Pathogenic Mutations and Responses to Zoledronic Acid in a Cohort of Osteogenesis Imperfecta Children. J Clin Endocrinol Metab 2022;107(9):2571–9.

26. Anam EA, Rauch F, Glorieux FH, et al. Osteotomy Healing in Children With Osteogenesis Imperfecta Receiving Bisphosphonate Treatment. J Bone Miner Res 2015;30(8):1362–8.

27. Munns CF, Rauch F, Zeitlin L, et al. Delayed osteotomy but not fracture healing in pediatric osteogenesis imperfecta patients receiving pamidronate. J Bone Miner Res 2004;19(11):1779–86.

28. Azzam KA, Rush ET, Burke BR, et al. Mid-term Results of Femoral and Tibial Osteotomies and Fassier-Duval Nailing in Children With Osteogenesis Imperfecta. J Pediatr Orthop 2018;38(6):331–6.

29. Holmes K, Gralla J, Brazell C, et al. Fassier-Duval Rod Failure: Is It Related to Positioning in the Distal Epiphysis? J Pediatr Orthop 2020;40(8):448–52.

30. el-Sobky MA, Hanna AA, Basha NE, et al. Surgery versus surgery plus pamidronate in the management of osteogenesis imperfecta patients: a comparative study. J Pediatr Orthop B 2006;15(3): 222–8.

31. Sabharwal S. Enhancement of bone formation during distraction osteogenesis: pediatric applications. J Am Acad Orthop Surg 2011;19(2):101–11.

32. Kiely P, Ward K, Bellemore CM, et al. Bisphosphonate rescue in distraction osteogenesis: a case series. J Pediatr Orthop 2007;27(4):467–71.

33. Vuorimies I, Toiviainen-Salo S, Hero M, et al. Zoledronic acid treatment in children with osteogenesis imperfecta. Horm Res Paediatr 2011;75(5):346–53.

34. Simm PJ, Biggin A, Zacharin MR, et al. Consensus guidelines on the use of bisphosphonate therapy in children and adolescents. J Paediatr Child Health 2018;54(3):223–33.

35. Munns CF, Rajab MH, Hong J, et al. Acute phase response and mineral status following low dose intravenous zoledronic acid in children. Bone 2007;41(3):366–70.

36. Black DM, Kelly MP, Genant HK, et al. Bisphosphonates and fractures of the subtrochanteric or diaphyseal femur. N Engl J Med 2010;362(19):1761–71.

37. Black DM, Geiger EJ, Eastell R, et al. Atypical Femur Fracture Risk versus Fragility Fracture Prevention with Bisphosphonates. N Engl J Med 2020; 383(8):743–53.

38. Trejo P, Fassier F, Glorieux FH, et al. Diaphyseal Femur Fractures in Osteogenesis Imperfecta: Characteristics and Relationship With Bisphosphonate Treatment. J Bone Miner Res 2017;32(5):1034–9.

39. Brown JJ, Ramalingam L, Zacharin MR. Bisphosphonate-associated osteonecrosis of the jaw: does it occur in children? Clin Endocrinol 2008;68(6):863–7.

40. Contaldo M, Luzzi V, Ierardo G, et al. Bisphosphonate-related osteonecrosis of the jaws and dental surgery procedures in children and young people with osteogenesis imperfecta: A systematic review.

J Stomatol Oral Maxillofac Surg 2020;121(5): 556–62.

41. Neal TW, Schlieve T. Medication-Related Osteonecrosis of the Jaws in the Pediatric Population. J Oral Maxillofac Surg 2022;80(10):1686–90.

42. Lozano-Calderon SA, Colman MW, Raskin KA, et al. Use of bisphosphonates in orthopedic surgery: pearls and pitfalls. Orthop Clin N Am 2014;45(3): 403–16.

43. Harding AK, Toksvig-Larsen S, Tagil M, et al. A single dose zoledronic acid enhances pin fixation in high tibial osteotomy using the hemicallotasis technique. A double-blind placebo controlled randomized study in 46 patients. Bone 2010;46(3): 649–54.

44. Liu B, Liu X, Chen Y, et al. Clinical effect observation of intravenous application of zoledronic acid in patients with cervical spondylosis and osteoporosis after anterior cervical discectomy and fusion: A randomized controlled study. J Orthop Surg 2019;27(2). 2309499019847028.

45. Cheng SH, Kuo YJ, Chen C, et al. Effects of teriparatide and bisphosphonate on spinal fusion procedure: A systematic review and network meta-analysis. PLoS One 2020;15(9):e0237566.

46. Ralston SH, Gaston MS. Management of Osteogenesis Imperfecta. Front Endocrinol 2019;10:924.

47. Lewiecki EM, Bilezikian JP, Giangregorio L, et al. Proceedings of the 2018 Santa Fe Bone Symposium: Advances in the Management of Osteoporosis. J Clin Densitom 2019;22(1):1–19.

48. Mugge L, DeBacker Dang D, Caras A, et al. Osteoporosis as a Risk Factor for Intraoperative Complications and Long-term Instrumentation Failure in Patients With Scoliotic Spinal Deformity. Spine 2022;47(20):1435–42.

Hand and Wrist

Surgical Considerations for Osteoporosis, Osteopenia, and Vitamin D Deficiency in Upper Extremity Surgery

Paul T. Greenfield, MD, Tori J. Coble, DO,
Jared A. Bell, MD, James H. Calandruccio, MD,
William J. Weller, MD*

KEYWORDS

• Osteoporosis • Osteopenia • Surgical considerations • Upper extremity • Fragility fractures
• Vitamin D deficiency • Bone health • Fracture prevention

KEY POINTS

- Osteoporosis, osteopenia, and vitamin D deficiency-related injuries in the upper extremity are common and are anticipated to rise with an aging population.
- During the perioperative period, it is important to identify the causes of low bone mineral density and initiate appropriate therapy.
- Fragility fractures can be challenging to treat surgically and necessitate special intraoperative considerations.
- The focus of postoperative management should be on preventing additional fractures through a healthy balance of diet, exercise, and medical therapy.

INTRODUCTION

Osteoporosis is characterized by disruption of bony architecture leading to deterioration of bone quality and loss of bone mass. Approximately 10 million people aged over 50 years are affected by osteoporosis.[1] Osteopenia, the precursor to osteoporosis, affects an additional 34 million Americans.[2] Vitamin D plays a direct role in bone health by promoting regulation of calcium and phosphate, both of which are essential elements for bone matrix integrity.[3] Deficiency leads to decreased bone mineral density (BMD), altered bone biomechanical properties, and increased fracture rates similar to osteoporosis and osteopenia.[4–6]

Osteopenia, osteoporosis, and vitamin D deficiency play a significant role in the prevalence, severity, and subsequent management of upper extremity injuries. It is well established that upper extremity fractures are directly correlated with decreased BMD. The incidence of fractures resulting from osteoporosis, often referred to as fragility fractures, exceeds 1.5 million in the United States alone.[1] The risk of sustaining a proximal humerus fracture increases 2.6 times in patients with osteoporotic bone versus nonosteoporotic bone.[7] Distal radius fractures in the elderly population may be the first clinical sign of osteoporosis and tend to be more severe than fractures in patients with normal BMD.[8,9] Patients with low BMD, therefore, require additional considerations that must be addressed during management of upper extremity injuries. Additional preoperative planning, differing operative techniques, and variable postoperative outcomes are all important factors for surgeons to understand in this population.

Hand and Wrist Section of *Orthopedic Clinics of North America*, Campbell Clinic Department of Orthopedic Surgery and Biomedical Engineering, University of Tennessee Health Science Center, 7887 Wolf River Boulevard, Germantown, TN 38138, USA
* Corresponding author.
E-mail address: wweller@campbellclinic.com

Orthop Clin N Am 55 (2024) 355–362
https://doi.org/10.1016/j.ocl.2024.02.005
0030-5898/24/

The purpose of this article is to review osteoporosis, osteopenia, and vitamin D deficiency within the scope of upper extremity surgery. We present a concise overview of the causes of low BMD and their clinical manifestations as they relate to upper extremity surgery. Additionally, we discuss preoperative testing, screening methodologies, nuanced intraoperative surgical techniques, and postoperative considerations tailored to this unique patient population.

NATURE OF THE PROBLEM
Osteoporosis and Osteopenia

Bone health is important in preventing the morbidity and mortality associated with fractures, especially in the rapidly growing elderly population. The strength of bone is largely determined by BMD.[10] Deterioration of bone at a cellular level leads to a loss of BMD and an increased susceptibility to fracture.[1] This deterioration is caused by an imbalance between osteoclast and osteoblast activity leading to an increased bone turnover.[2,10] As bone turnover increases, BMD decreases, eventually leading to osteopenia and osteoporosis. Osteopenia is defined by the World Health Organization as a BMD T-score greater than −2.5 but less than −1 as measured by dual-energy x-ray absorptiometric (DEXA) scan. Osteoporosis is the more severe form of the disease and includes patients with T-scores less than −2.5.[2]

Multiple risk factors exist for developing osteoporosis and osteopenia. Women, particularly after menopause, are 4 times more likely than men to develop osteopenia.[2] This is largely due to the protective effects of progesterone and estrogen on bone health. After menopause, the decrease in these hormones leads to a decrease in BMD and eventually osteopenia and osteoporosis.[11] Other nonmodifiable risk factors include age, race, and genetics.[5] Modifiable risk factors include alcohol use, smoking status, and activity level. While bone mass naturally begins to decline after the age of 30 years, these risk factors can accelerate the loss of BMD and lead to osteopenia and osteoporosis. Identifying these risk factors allows for appropriate consultation with patients on various interventions to address them.

Vitamin D Deficiency

Bone is metabolically active and undergoes continuous remodeling through the interplay of multiple trace elements, nutrients, and hormones. Two of the most important trace elements contributing to BMD are calcium and phosphorus.[11] Vitamin D, also known as calciferol, plays a pivotal role in calcium and phosphorus homeostasis. Vitamin D is synthesized in the skin from its precursors following ultraviolet B photon exposure. It directly affects intestinal absorption and urinary secretion of calcium and phosphorus.[6] Low vitamin D levels ultimately lead to decreased serum calcium levels, which have been identified as a risk factor for low BMD as it leads to increased bone resorption.[11] Deficiency is defined by the National Academy of Medicine as serum levels of 25-hydroxycholecalciferol less than 12 ng/mL, while levels of 12 to 20 ng/mL are adequate to maintain bone health.[12] Vitamin D levels should be regularly checked to ensure appropriate levels and appropriately address a modifiable risk factor of low BMD.

CLINICAL RELEVANCE

The biomechanical changes to bone caused by osteoporosis, osteopenia, and vitamin D deficiency play an important role in fracture prevalence, severity, and outcomes. Upper extremity fractures are very common with an incidence of 67.7 fractures per 10,000 people in the United States. Of these, distal radius fractures are the most common at 16.2 fractures per 10,000 people and proximal humerus fractures are third at 6 fractures per 10,000 people. Distal radius fractures are bimodal in distribution, with a large portion of fractures occurring in people aged over 65 years.[13] Wrist fractures in the elderly population are often caused by a fall onto an outstretched arm and have long been regarded as a classic osteoporotic fragility fracture.[14] These fractures can serve as sentinel events before other fragility fractures such as hip and vertebral fractures.[15–17] By 2025, it is predicted that more than 3 million osteoporotic fractures will incur a cost of over US$25 billion in the United States alone.[18] Women account for the majority of these fractures, incurring a lifetime risk of any osteoporotic fracture of 40% to 50% compared to 13% to 42% for men.[19] As medical treatments and lifestyle continue to improve and the older population continues to grow, the surgical treatment of upper extremity fractures in patients with diminished bone quality will play a larger role in orthopedic hand and upper extremity surgery.

Treatment of upper extremity fractures in patients with fragility fractures differs from patients with normal BMD. As patients age and BMD decreases, the load to failure decreases.[20,21] Older patients sustain fractures from low-energy trauma and resultant forces that would normally not cause injury in patients with a normal BMD. Not only are patients with osteopenia, osteoporosis, and vitamin D deficiency more prone to fractures but also the fractures that do occur tend to be more severe.[8,20] Clayton and colleagues[8] showed that patients with osteoporosis suffered more severe, intra-articular distal radius fractures than age-matched patients with normal BMD. Additionally, it is more difficult to assess the severity of these injuries with conventional x-ray due to the lower BMD. Lill and colleagues[20] showed that the severity of distal radius fractures in patients with osteopenia is often underestimated on conventional plain films. These additional factors add increased complexity to presurgical planning and should be considered prior to undergoing surgical intervention for upper extremity fractures in patients with low BMD.

Osteopenia, osteoporosis, and vitamin D deficiency not only affect fracture prevalence and severity but also play an important role in long-term outcomes and mortality. Wrist fractures are often seen in older patients who have enough coordination to attempt to break a ground level fall with an outstretched arm.[22] They are often the first in a series of frailty injuries to occur and can be an indicator of future disability and mortality. Edwards and colleagues[23] found that women with osteoporosis who suffered a wrist fracture were 50% more likely to have a clinically important functional decline. Rozental and colleagues[24] also found that mortality rate increased by 14% only 7 years after patients aged over 65 years suffered a distal radius fracture. Additionally, elderly men were twice as likely to die and did so in half the time as compared to elderly women who suffered a distal radius fracture. Additionally, patients with osteoporosis who undergo open reduction and internal fixation of a distal radius fracture have higher Disability of the Arm, Shoulder, and Hand scores by 15 points compared to patients without osteoporosis.[25] These outcomes are important for orthopedic surgeons to understand when evaluating and treating fractures of the upper extremity in patients with low BMD.

DISCUSSION
Perioperative Management
The orthopedic surgeon is usually introduced to the patient and their care team following an initial injury. Due to the time-sensitive nature of fracture management, it is neither always possible nor required to screen for low BMD prior to treatment. Ideally, the management of patients with low BMD begins with their primary care physician after a screening test and not after sustaining a fragility fracture. Unfortunately, this is not always the case, and it is recommended that the patient be counseled and follow-up scheduled with their primary care team in the perioperative period for a proper evaluation and discussion of long-term management. The typical workup should include a combination of BMD testing, assessment tools, and laboratory work. It is recommended that all patients with upper extremity fragility fractures undergo screening with BMD testing.[26] DEXA scan at the hip and lumbar spine stands as the current gold standard for detecting low BMD. The Fracture Risk Assessment Tool (FRAX) is also a useful screening tool for physicians to identify patients at risk for subsequent osteoporotic fracture. This is particularly helpful in frailty fractures of the upper extremity, as these are often considered sentinel fractures as mentioned earlier. Many studies have shown that most patients are not effectively evaluated for low BMD following a fragility fracture, and this is a key component in future management and prevention.[17,27]

Patients should also be evaluated for correctable causes of secondary osteoporosis, osteopenia, and vitamin D deficiency. This involves laboratory testing of a basic metabolic panel, complete blood count, calcium, 25-hydroxy vitamin D, parathyroid hormone (PTH), and thyroid-stimulating hormone levels.[17,22,28] When appropriate, a referral may be necessary to an endocrinologist for correction of metabolic derangements such as hypercalcemia or hypocalcemia. Endocrinology referral is also recommended when patients have had more than 2 fragility fractures, have a contraindication to bisphosphonate treatment, or sustain a frailty fracture after receiving bisphosphonates for over 5 years.[28] Current guidelines from the National Osteoporosis Foundation (NOF) recommend 1200 mg of calcium per day for women over 50 years and men over 70 years.[26] It is important to note that larger calcium intakes (1500–2000 mg/d) are associated with elevated cardiovascular risk and should be avoided.[29] Recommendations also suggest both men and women aged over 50 years intake 800 to 1000 IU/d of vitamin D3.[26] Ensuring patients have adequate perioperative metabolic levels aids not only in postoperative healing but also in the prevention of future fragility fractures.

Bisphosphonates are the first-line recommendation when pharmacologic treatment is warranted based on preoperative DEXA and FRAX screening. NOF guidelines recommend bisphosphonate treatment in all patients with a T-score less than −2.5 measured by DEXA scanning.[26] Additionally, postmenopausal women and men aged over 50 years with low BMD (T-score between −1.0 and −2.5) measured by DEXA and a 10 year hip fracture probability greater than 3% based on FRAX screening should also be started on bisphosphonates. Other Food and Drug Administration-approved pharmacologic options include selective estrogen receptor modulators, calcitonin, recombinant PTH, and receptor activator of nuclear factor kappa-B ligand inhibitors.[17] It is important for the primary or endocrinology team to initiate treatment in order to monitor patients closely on these therapies as long-term treatment is not advised given their risk profiles when taken for extended periods.

Finally, modifiable lifestyle factors should be discussed and appropriately addressed. It is important to minimize the risk of falls and future fractures while also encouraging activities that promote balance, strength, and coordination. Gillespie and colleagues[30] found that group and home-based exercises programs reduce the rates of falling among older adults living in the community. Tai Chi has been shown to not only reduce falls but may also attenuate loss of BMD in women with osteopenia.[30,31] Polypharmacy is also very common in older patients.[22] Avoiding medications with central nervous system depressive effects and judicious use of antihypertensives can also aid in minimizing fall risk.[26] Overall, patients with low BMD should be treated surgically when appropriate and referred to a primary care provider for a multidisciplinary approach focused on appropriate screening and both pharmacologic and lifestyle therapies.

Intraoperative Management

Intraoperative and postoperative considerations for the treatment of upper extremity fractures in patients on the osteoporosis spectrum are crucial for optimal outcomes and mitigating associated complications. Proximal humerus and distal radius fractures due to a low-energy mechanism are the 2 most common surgical pathologies seen in these populations.[32–34] While many concepts discussed here are directed toward those injuries, the principles are often applicable to other osteoporotic fractures of the upper extremity.

In many cases, a conventional open treatment is necessary to achieve adequate exposure and fixation. However, where a minimally invasive technique can be utilized while still achieving an appropriate reduction and fixation, this can lead to decreased soft tissue and periosteal disruption.[35] Minimally invasive plate

osteosynthesis (MIPO) for proximal humerus and distal radius fractures may lead to improved functional outcome, range of motion, postoperative pain, and/or patient satisfaction when compared to conventional methods.[36–40] However, caution should be exercised when considering MIPO, as it is not recommended for intra-articular fracture patterns.[41] Intramedullary nails for extra-articular distal radius and proximal humerus fractures can also be considered. They have been shown to offer equivalent improvements in functional and radiographic outcomes when compared to plate fixation but are not commonly utilized for distal radius fractures.[42,43] The use of reverse total shoulder and total elbow arthroplasty has been increasing as treatment options for older individuals with complex, displaced osteoporotic fractures, yielding promising results.[44–48] Finally, external fixation or spanning devices that rely on ligamentotaxis can be considered in highly comminuted fracture patterns, resulting in acceptable radiographic results and functional outcomes.[49]

Fortunately, there are implant options designed specifically to address low BMD in fracture fixation. Screw mechanics are essential, as BMD is directly correlated to screw purchase. Cancellous screws, with their increased outer diameter and pitch, have demonstrated greater stiffness and pullout strength compared to cortical screws in osteoporotic bone.[50] These benefits diminish when the BMD drops below 0.4 g/cm^3.[51] The advent of locking plate technology, which does not rely on the friction between the bone and plate, has significantly enhanced the fixation strength of constructs used to treat fragility fractures. These fixed-angle devices do not necessitate strong metaphyseal bone for implant stability, making them excellent options for osteoporotic bone fixation.[52–54] Choosing an implant with a divergent screw pattern has also proven to boost the stability of the construct, reducing the chances of fixation loss.[55] At times, the use of dual plating might be suitable, providing robust fixation without relying solely on a single plate. This method has been well studied for osteoporotic fractures of the lower extremities with positive outcomes, but there is limited yet recent evidence for its applicability to certain osteoporotic fractures of the upper extremities.[56–60] Seok and colleagues[61] noted improved neck-shaft angles on radiographs and better functional outcome scores in the dual-plated proximal humerus cohort when compared to the lateral locking plate group.

In instances of significant bone loss or impaction, implants can be reinforced with bone and biologic augmentation to boost stability. Common options include polymethyl methacrylate (PMMA), bone substitutes, and bone grafts. Augmentation with PMMA or calcium phosphate can be performed by introducing or injecting them into the metaphyseal bone in combination with locking plate fixation, reducing the risk of cutout and increasing the load to failure.[62–64] Calcium phosphate boasts advantages over PMMA since it does not undergo an exothermic reaction, which might cause thermal damage to surrounding osteocytes, and it gets absorbed as new bone forms.[64] Calcium sulfate, another bone substitute, has a faster absorption period, roughly 8 weeks, which might be more or less favorable than calcium phosphate, which takes months to years based on the quantity used.[65] Bone autograft or allograft, such as a fibular strut allograft or cancellous iliac crest autograft, is a viable option. The fibular strut has been described to reinforce the medial column of the proximal humerus[66,67] and iliac crest autograft can facilitate fracture healing with good results, although typically reserved for nonunions.[68]

Postoperative Management

After surgical fixation of a fragility fracture, postoperative care encompasses early range of motion and rehabilitation. Bracing may be necessary until the fracture has completely healed. Once the fracture has healed, the primary emphasis shifts to preventing future fractures. This prevention strategy includes endorsing weight-bearing exercises, balance training, resuming appropriate medications to boost BMD, maintaining a nutritious diet, and re-establishing regular follow-ups with a multidisciplinary team, including a primary care physician and specialists like rheumatologists, endocrinologists, or geriatricians, as previously mentioned.[22,69]

SUMMARY

Osteoporosis, osteopenia, and vitamin D deficiency pose a significant and challenging role in the surgical treatment of upper extremity fractures. As the elderly population continues to grow, the number of low-energy fragility fractures is expected to increase as well. These patients, having compromised bone health with impaired healing potential, subsequently require specialized care. This study highlights the importance of a timely surgical evaluation as well as a referral to a multidisciplinary team of primary care providers, endocrinologists, and geriatricians to assess patients for low BMD and identify medical treatments in conjunction with surgical treatment when indicated. Such assessment includes appropriate screening with DEXA, as well as the initiation of both pharmaceutical and lifestyle therapies. Additionally, surgical considerations to treat low BMD and minimize complications comprise varying techniques, implant designs, and augmentation to create a stable construct amidst compromised bone quality. Early postoperative motion and rehabilitation are encouraged. Prioritizing future fracture prevention through patient education and a multifaceted approach is key to improving healing and preventing morbidity and mortality in this vulnerable population.

CLINICS CARE POINTS

- Upper extremity fractures due to low BMD can be caused by osteopenia, osteoporosis, and vitamin D deficiency and are increasing in prevalence as the aging population increases.
- Fragility fractures of the upper extremity require a multidisciplinary approach to care including appropriate screening and treatment by primary care providers, geriatricians, endocrinologists, and orthopedic surgeons.
- Cancellous screws, locking plates, and biologic augmentation are all useful tools for increasing fixation construct strength in patients with low BMD.
- Postoperative care for patients with fragility fractures of the upper extremity should focus on early range of motion, rehabilitation, and prevention of future fractures through a multifaceted approach.

DISCLOSURE

The authors have nothing to disclose.

REFERENCES

1. Clynes MA, Harvey NC, Curtis EM, et al. The epidemiology of osteoporosis. Br Med Bull 2020;133(1): 105–17.
2. Varacallo M, Seaman TJ, Jandu JS, et al. Osteopenia, in StatPearls. Treasure Island (FL): StatPearls Publishing Copyright © 2023, StatPearls Publishing LLC; 2023.
3. Entezari V, Lazarus M. Surgical Considerations in Managing Osteoporosis, Osteopenia, and Vitamin D Deficiency During Arthroscopic Rotator Cuff Repair. Orthop Clin N Am 2019;50(2):233–43.

4. Bouillon R, Carmeliet G. Vitamin D insufficiency: Definition, diagnosis and management. Best Pract Res Clin Endocrinol Metabol 2018;32(5):669–84.

5. Tański W, Kosiorowska J, Szymańska-Chabowska A. Osteoporosis - risk factors, pharmaceutical and non-pharmaceutical treatment. Eur Rev Med Pharmacol Sci 2021;25(9):3557–66.

6. Janoušek J, Pilařová V, Macáková K, et al. Vitamin D: sources, physiological role, biokinetics, deficiency, therapeutic use, toxicity, and overview of analytical methods for detection of vitamin D and its metabolites. Crit Rev Clin Lab Sci 2022;59(8):517–54.

7. Stone MA, Namdari S. Surgical Considerations in the Treatment of Osteoporotic Proximal Humerus Fractures. Orthop Clin N Am 2019;50(2):223–31.

8. Clayton RA, Gaston MS, Ralston SH, et al. Association between decreased bone mineral density and severity of distal radial fractures. J Bone Joint Surg Am 2009;91(3):613–9.

9. Wu JC, Strickland CD, Chambers JS. Wrist Fractures and Osteoporosis. Orthop Clin N Am 2019;50(2):211–21.

10. Lane NE. Epidemiology, etiology, and diagnosis of osteoporosis. Am J Obstet Gynecol 2006;194(2 Suppl):S3–11.

11. Ciosek Ż, Kot K, Kosik-Bogacka D, et al. The Effects of Calcium, Magnesium, Phosphorus, Fluoride, and Lead on Bone Tissue. Biomolecules 2021;11(4):506.

12. LeFevre ML, LeFevre NM. Vitamin D Screening and Supplementation in Community-Dwelling Adults: Common Questions and Answers. Am Fam Physician 2018;97(4):254–60.

13. Karl JW, Olson PR, Rosenwasser MP. The Epidemiology of Upper Extremity Fractures in the United States, 2009. J Orthop Trauma 2015;29(8):e242-4.

14. Cummings SR, Melton LJ. Epidemiology and outcomes of osteoporotic fractures. Lancet 2002;359(9319):1761–7.

15. Cuddihy MT, Gabriel SE, Crowson CS, et al. Forearm fractures as predictors of subsequent osteoporotic fractures. Osteoporos Int 1999;9(6):469–75.

16. Ostergaard PJ, Hall MJ, Rozental TD. Considerations in the Treatment of Osteoporotic Distal Radius Fractures in Elderly Patients. Current Reviews in Musculoskeletal Medicine 2019;12(1):50–6.

17. Shoji MM, Ingall EM, Rozental TD. Upper Extremity Fragility Fractures. J Hand Surg Am 2021;46(2):126–32.

18. Burge R, Dawson-Hughes B, Solomon DH, et al. Incidence and economic burden of osteoporosis-related fractures in the United States, 2005-2025. J Bone Miner Res 2007;22(3):465–75.

19. Johnell O, Kanis J. Epidemiology of osteoporotic fractures. Osteoporos Int 2005;(16 Suppl 2):S3–7.

20. Lill CA, Goldhahn J, Albrecht A, et al. Impact of bone density on distal radius fracture patterns and comparison between five different fracture classifications. J Orthop Trauma 2003;17(4):271–8.

21. von Rüden C, Augat P. Failure of fracture fixation in osteoporotic bone. Injury 2016;(47 Suppl 2):S3–10.

22. Bukata SV, Kates SL, O'Keefe RJ. Short-term and long-term orthopaedic issues in patients with fragility fractures. Clin Orthop Relat Res 2011;469(8):2225–36.

23. Edwards BJ, Song J, Dunlop DD, et al. Functional decline after incident wrist fractures–Study of Osteoporotic Fractures: prospective cohort study. BMJ 2010;341:c3324.

24. Rozental TD, Branas CC, Bozentka DJ, et al. Survival among elderly patients after fractures of the distal radius. J Hand Surg Am 2002;27(6):948–52.

25. Fitzpatrick SK, Casemyr NE, Zurakowski D, et al. The effect of osteoporosis on outcomes of operatively treated distal radius fractures. J Hand Surg Am 2012;37(10):2027–34.

26. Cosman F, de Beur SJ, LeBoff MS, et al. Clinician's Guide to Prevention and Treatment of Osteoporosis. Osteoporos Int 2014;25(10):2359–81.

27. Rozental TD, Makhni EC, Day CS, et al. Improving evaluation and treatment for osteoporosis following distal radial fractures. A prospective randomized intervention. J Bone Joint Surg Am 2008;90(5):953–61.

28. Foote JE, Rozental TD. Osteoporosis and upper extremity fragility fractures. J Hand Surg Am 2012;37(1):165–7.

29. Bolland MJ, Grey AB, Gamble GD, et al. Effect of osteoporosis treatment on mortality: a meta-analysis. J Clin Endocrinol Metab 2010;95(3):1174–81.

30. Gillespie LD, Robertson MC, Gillespie WJ, et al. Interventions for preventing falls in older people living in the community. Cochrane Database Syst Rev 2012;2012(9):Cd007146.

31. Wayne PM, Kiel DP, Buring JE, et al. Impact of Tai Chi exercise on multiple fracture-related risk factors in post-menopausal osteopenic women: a pilot pragmatic, randomized trial. BMC Compl Alternative Med 2012;12:7.

32. Baron JA, Karagas M, Barrett J, et al. Basic epidemiology of fractures of the upper and lower limb among Americans over 65 years of age. Epidemiology 1996;7(6):612–8.

33. Chung KC, Shauver MJ, Birkmeyer JD. Trends in the United States in the treatment of distal radial fractures in the elderly. J Bone Joint Surg Am 2009;91(8):1868–73.

34. Court-Brown CM, Caesar B. Epidemiology of adult fractures: A review. Injury 2006;37(8):691–7.

35. García-Virto V, Santiago-Maniega S, Llorente-Peris A, et al. MIPO helical pre-contoured plates in diaphyseal humeral fractures with proximal extension. Surgical technique and results. Injury 2021;(52 Suppl 4):S125–30.

36. Bogner R, Hübner C, Matis N, et al. Minimally-invasive treatment of three- and four-part fractures of the proximal humerus in elderly patients. J Bone Joint Surg Br 2008;90(12):1602–7.

37. Buchmann L, van Lieshout EMM, Zeelenberg M, et al. Proximal humerus fractures (PHFs): comparison of functional outcome 1 year after minimally invasive plate osteosynthesis (MIPO) versus open reduction internal fixation (ORIF). Eur J Trauma Emerg Surg 2022;48(6):4553–8.

38. Kim JW, Oh CW, Byun YS, et al. A prospective randomized study of operative treatment for noncomminuted humeral shaft fractures: conventional open plating versus minimal invasive plate osteosynthesis. J Orthop Trauma 2015;29(4):189–94.

39. Lee DY, Park YJ, Park JS. A Meta-analysis of Studies of Volar Locking Plate Fixation of Distal Radius Fractures: Conventional versus Minimally Invasive Plate Osteosynthesis. Clin Orthop Surg 2019;11(2):208–19.

40. Li F, Liu X, Wang F, et al. Comparison between minimally invasive plate osteosynthesis and open reduction-internal fixation for proximal humeral fractures: a meta-analysis based on 1050 individuals. BMC Muscoskel Disord 2019;20(1):550.

41. Chen CY, Lin KC, Yang SW, et al. Clinical results of using minimally invasive long plate osteosynthesis versus conventional approach for extensive comminuted metadiaphyseal fractures of the radius. Arch Orthop Trauma Surg 2015;135(3):361–7.

42. Plate JF, Gaffney DL, Emory CL, et al. Randomized comparison of volar locking plates and intramedullary nails for unstable distal radius fractures. J Hand Surg Am 2015;40(6):1095–101.

43. Wang M, Wang X, Cai P, et al. Locking plate fixation versus intramedullary nail fixation for the treatment of multifragmentary proximal humerus fractures (OTA/AO type 11C): a preliminary comparison of clinical efficacy. BMC Muscoskel Disord 2023;24(1):461.

44. DeSimone LJ, Sanchez-Sotelo J. Total elbow arthroplasty for distal humerus fractures. Orthop Clin N Am 2013;44(3):381–7.

45. Egol KA, Tsai P, Vazques O, et al. Comparison of functional outcomes of total elbow arthroplasty vs plate fixation for distal humerus fractures in osteoporotic elbows. Am J Orthop (Belle Mead NJ) 2011;40(2):67–71.

46. Mata-Fink A, Meinke M, Jones C, et al. Reverse shoulder arthroplasty for treatment of proximal humeral fractures in older adults: a systematic review. J Shoulder Elbow Surg 2013;22(12):1737–48.

47. Rajaee SS, Yalamanchili D, Noori N, et al. Increasing Use of Reverse Total Shoulder Arthroplasty for Proximal Humerus Fractures in Elderly Patients. Orthopedics 2017;40(6):e982–9.

48. Schairer WW, Nwachukwu BU, Lyman S, et al. Arthroplasty treatment of proximal humerus fractures: 14-year trends in the United States. Phys Sportsmed 2017;45(2):92–6.

49. Vakhshori V, Alluri RK, Stevanovic M, et al. Review of Internal Radiocarpal Distraction Plating for Distal Radius Fracture Fixation. Hand (N Y) 2020;15(1):116–24.

50. Wang T, Boone C, Behn AW, et al. Cancellous Screws Are Biomechanically Superior to Cortical Screws in Metaphyseal Bone. Orthopedics 2016;39(5):e828–32.

51. Turner IG, Rice GN. Comparison of bone screw holding strength in healthy bovine and osteoporotic human cancellous bone. Clin Mater 1992;9(2):105–7.

52. Kralinger F, Blauth M, Goldhahn J, et al. The Influence of Local Bone Density on the Outcome of One Hundred and Fifty Proximal Humeral Fractures Treated with a Locking Plate. J Bone Joint Surg Am 2014;96(12):1026–32.

53. Omid R, Trasolini NA, Stone MA, et al. Principles of Locking Plate Fixation of Proximal Humerus Fractures. J Am Acad Orthop Surg 2021;29(11):e523–35.

54. Orbay JL, Fernandez DL. Volar fixed-angle plate fixation for unstable distal radius fractures in the elderly patient. J Hand Surg Am 2004;29(1):96–102.

55. Newman JM, Kahn M, Gruson KI. Reducing Postoperative Fracture Displacement After Locked Plating of Proximal Humerus Fractures: Current Concepts. Am J Orthop (Belle Mead NJ) 2015;44(7):312–20.

56. Choi S, Seo KB, Kwon YS, et al. Dual plate for comminuted proximal humerus fractures. Acta Orthop Belg 2019;85(4):429–36.

57. Rozell JC, Vemulapalli KC, Gary JL, et al. Tibial Plateau Fractures in Elderly Patients. Geriatr Orthop Surg Rehabil 2016;7(3):126–34.

58. Sanders R, Swiontkowski M, Rosen H, et al. Double-plating of comminuted, unstable fractures of the distal part of the femur. J Bone Joint Surg Am 1991;73(3):341–6.

59. Steinberg EL, Elis J, Steinberg Y, et al. A double-plating approach to distal femur fracture: A clinical study. Injury 2017;48(10):2260–5.

60. Ziran BH, Rohde RH, Wharton AR. Lateral and anterior plating of intra-articular distal femoral fractures treated via an anterior approach. Int Orthop 2002;26(6):370–3.

61. Seok HG, Park SG. Dual plate fixation for proximal humerus fractures with unstable medial column in patients with osteoporosis: A case-control study. J Orthop Trauma 2023;37(10):e387–93.

62. Cameron HU, Jacob R, Macnab I, et al. Use of polymethylmethacrylate to enhance screw fixation in bone. J Bone Joint Surg Am 1975;57(5):655–6.

63. Jaeblon T. Polymethylmethacrylate: properties and contemporary uses in orthopaedics. J Am Acad Orthop Surg 2010;18(5):297–305.

64. Larsson S, Stadelmann VA, Arnoldi J, et al. Injectable calcium phosphate cement for augmentation

around cancellous bone screws. In vivo biomechanical studies. J Biomech 2012;45(7):1156–60.

65. Tay BK, Patel VV, Bradford DS. Calcium sulfate- and calcium phosphate-based bone substitutes. Mimicry of the mineral phase of bone. Orthop Clin N Am 1999;30(4):615–23.

66. Bae JH, Oh JK, Chon CS, et al. The biomechanical performance of locking plate fixation with intramedullary fibular strut graft augmentation in the treatment of unstable fractures of the proximal humerus. J Bone Joint Surg Br 2011;93(7):937–41.

67. Chow RM, Begum F, Beaupre LA, et al. Proximal humeral fracture fixation: locking plate construct ± intramedullary fibular allograft. J Shoulder Elbow Surg 2012;21(7):894–901.

68. Zhu L, Liu Y, Yang Z, et al. Locking plate fixation combined with iliac crest bone autologous graft for proximal humerus comminuted fracture. Chin Med J (Engl) 2014;127(9):1672–6.

69. Benedetti MG, Furlini G, Zati A, et al. The Effectiveness of Physical Exercise on Bone Density in Osteoporotic Patients. BioMed Res Int 2018;2018:4840531.

Shoulder and Elbow

A Systematic Review of Patient Selection Criteria for Outpatient Total Shoulder Arthroplasty

Kevin T. Root, BS[a], Keegan M. Hones, MD, MS[b],
Kevin A. Hao, BS[a], Tyler J. Brolin, MD[c],
Jonathan O. Wright, MD[b], Joseph J. King, MD[b],
Thomas W. Wright, MD[b], Bradley S. Schoch, MD[d],*

KEYWORDS

- Shoulder arthroplasty • Total shoulder arthroplasty • TSA • Outpatient • Patient selection

KEY POINTS

- There is no single set of accepted patient selection criteria for outpatient TSA. Here, the authors identify and systematically review available literature to propose evidence-based criteria that merit postoperative admission.
- The surveyed literature indicates that patients with a limited ability to ambulate independently or a history of congestive heart failure should be admitted postoperatively for monitoring unless otherwise cleared for discharge.
- In addition, age 85+, renal insufficiency, poorly controlled diabetes mellitus, and a positive smoking status were identified as risk factors with varying levels of significance for increased LOS or early adverse events.

INTRODUCTION

The utilization of total shoulder arthroplasty (TSA) increased by 103% between 2011 and 2017 and is projected to outpace the growth rate of total hip arthroplasty and total knee arthroplasty through 2025.[1] The annual health care costs are projected to range up to $1.8 billion, emphasizing the need to maximize value-based care on behalf of providers and patients.[2] Several studies have demonstrated that opting for outpatient over inpatient TSA may provide a solution by reducing costs while maintaining or improving patient outcomes and satisfaction.[3–8]

Brolin and colleagues conducted a survey of active American Shoulder and Elbow Surgeon members to identify barriers to the adoption of routine outpatient TSA.[9] Identified barriers included patient selection factors such as comorbidities, patient support systems, medical complication, and risk of readmission.[4,5,7,9–17] Despite these perceived barriers, previous studies have demonstrated, with appropriate patient selection; TSA can be performed in an outpatient setting while maintaining equivocal or superior patient safety and outcomes.[3,5,11,12,18] It is therefore essential for surgeons to be familiar with proper patient selection criteria when recommending outpatient TSA. Identified risk factors

---

[a] College of Medicine, University of Florida, 1600 SW Archer Road, Gainesville, FL 32610, USA; [b] Department of Orthopaedics and Sports Medicine, University of Florida, 3450 Hull Road # 3341, Gainesville, FL 32607, USA; [c] Department of Orthopaedic Surgery, University of Tennessee-Campbell Clinic, 1211 Union Avenue # 500, Memphis, TN 38104, USA; [d] Department of Orthopedic Surgery, Mayo Clinic, 4500 San Pablo Road, Jacksonville, FL 32224, USA
* Corresponding author.
E-mail address: Schoch.bradley@mayo.edu

Orthop Clin N Am 55 (2024) 363–381
https://doi.org/10.1016/j.ocl.2023.12.002

that predispose patients to requiring an increased length of patient stay or complications include age, sex, body mass index (BMI), race, ability to ambulate independently, smoking status, comorbidities, opioid consumption, steroid use, and depression.[19-28] However, there is no single set of accepted criteria, and patient selection criteria continue to evolve as new evidence becomes available.

Owing to a lack of universally accepted criteria, the onus is on the surgeon to review the literature and apply it to their clinical practice. In this regard, the purpose of this review is foremost to highlight documented risk factors for extended length of stay (LOS), complications, and readmission after TSA. In addition, the authors proposed evidence-based criteria that merit postoperative admission.

METHODS

Eligibility Criteria

The authors included studies according to the following eligibility criteria, based on population/patient/problem, comparison/control, intervention/exposure, outcome (PICO).

1. Population: Patients undergoing orthopedic surgery for joint pathology
2. Intervention/exposure: Shoulder arthroplasty (anatomic TSA [aTSA] and reverse TSA [rTSA])
3. Characteristic/outcomes: LOS, surgical complications, and readmission rates
4. Study design: The authors included case-control, cross-sectional studies, and systematic reviews.

Search Strategy and Study Selection

In accordance with Preferred Reporting Items for Systematic Reviews and Meta-Analyses (PRISMA),[29] a systematic search of the literature was performed (Supplement 1). The authors queried PubMed/MEDLINE, Embase, and Cochrane databases from inception until June 1, 2022, to identify articles written in the English language on outpatient TSA as defined as Ambulatory Surgery[30] or looking at same-day discharge (<23 hour stay) per the billing definition or both.

Search terms included "total shoulder arthroplasty," "TSA," "shoulder arthroplasty," "outpatient," "same-day," "patient selection," "optimal candidate," "contraindication," "risk factor," "safe," and "satisfactory." Studies were excluded from: only addressing outpatient TSA, not including outcomes of interest, sample size less then n = 10, and not written in English. Titles and abstracts were screened by one author (KTR). Subsequently, full texts of the remaining articles

were reviewed, which was performed by one author (KTR). The full text of relevant papers was retrieved, and references of relevant reviews or original articles were investigated to identify further eligible studies. Included studies were approved by the senior author.

Data Extraction and Synthesis

For each included study, the following factors were recorded: author name, publication year, level of scientific evidence, sample size, and breakdown. Clinical outcomes recorded were risk factors associated with increased LOS; increased readmission; revision rate; decreased chance of same-day discharge; and increased postsurgery morbidity, mortality, or complication. Risk factors investigated include age, BMI, sex, race, patient independence, patient support system, patient functional status, and patient ability to ambulate independently American Society of Anesthesiology (ASA) score, Charlson–Deyo index score, smoking status, patient medications, and patient comorbidities.

The database and manual search identified 107 unique articles following duplicate exclusion. Sixty-one articles were excluded during title and abstract screening, leaving 46 articles for full-text review. Full-text screening led to the inclusion of 14 articles[8,9,12,19-21,23,25-27] (Fig. 1). A narrative review of the available studies was then performed.

RESULTS

Study Characteristics

The 14 articles included in the analysis reported on 521,168 TSAs. Of the 14 included articles, all were authored in either the United States (13/14, 93%) or Qatar (1/14, 7%). Of these, 2/14 (13%) were systematic reviews,[10,11] 7/14 (50%) were retrospective studies,[12,21,22,24,26-28] 2/14 (14%) were epidemiology studies,[23,31] 1/14 (7%) was a therapeutic study,[19] 1/14 (7%) was a predictive model study,[20] and 1/14 (7%) was a database analysis.[25]

Age

Age is a key factor in outpatient TSA patient selection. In a recent study, Cimino and colleagues[5] found outpatient (Ambulatory Surgery) TSA candidates to be 3.4 years younger on average (66.6 vs 70 years). However, TSA is increasingly performed in patients above the age of 70 years in both settings.[32] Older age has been broadly associated with increased LOS, risk of readmission, surgical complications, and mortality.[20,23-25] In patients ≥65 year old who underwent aTSA or rTSA under a single

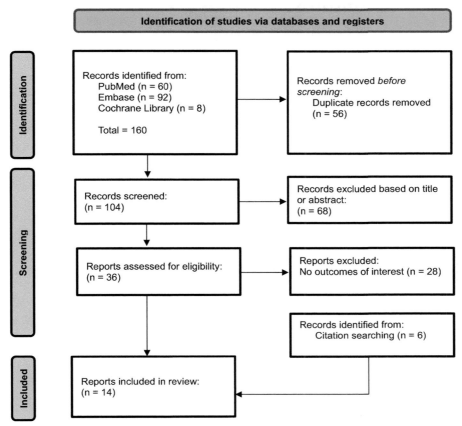

Fig. 1. Preferred Reporting Items for Systematic Reviews and Meta-Analyses (PRISMA) flow diagram depicting article identification, subsequent exclusion, and analysis.

surgeon, Willenbring and colleagues[28] found a 1-year increase in age increased the odds of a postoperative surgical complication up to 1 year after surgery, irrespective of surgical setting. Waterman and colleagues[27] conducted a retrospective cohort study of primary unilateral aTSA and rTSA and found increasing age to be an independent predictor of mortality (OR 1.19; 95% CI, 1.06–1.33) and a near twofold increase in mortality odds for every 10 years of life. Although these studies demonstrate that greater age is associated with an increased predisposition of morbidity and mortality after TSA, they do not provide evidence to support an age cutoff whereby the risk of adverse events increases non-linearly, specifically in the immediate postoperative period. However, other studies have attempted to compare old and young patients undergoing TSA in an outpatient versus inpatient setting to identify a threshold. In a retrospective cohort study of 123,347 Medicare subscribers who underwent aTSA or rTSA in an inpatient or outpatient (Ambulatory Surgery) setting, Basques and colleagues[12] found

an increased rate of (re)admission after outpatient TSA for those 85 years or older (OR = 34.1, $P < .001$). In addition, in an analysis of 2004 inpatient, primary unilateral aTSAs, Dunn and colleagues[23] found advanced age ($\geq$80 years vs <60 years) to be associated with increased LOS (OR = 2.13; 95% CI, 1.11–4.07; $P = .011$). In patients receiving an elective aTSA or rTSA in an outpatient setting (Ambulatory Surgery), Carbone and colleagues[22] found the age 80 to 85 years group to have an increased risk of 90-day all-cause (re)admission (OR 3.46; 95% CI, 1.75–6.85; $P<.001$). Based on the available evidence, patient age $\geq$80 years may be an indication for admission after TSA. However, additional research directly comparing complications, readmission, and increased LOS after outpatient versus inpatient TSA in different age groups is needed (Table 1).

Body Mass Index
BMI is associated with increased (re)admission and complication rates.[10,11,24] The association between BMI and LOS has been studied and is

Table 1
Summary of literature evaluating the influence of patient age on eligibility for outpatient total shoulder arthroplasty

Author et al (Year)	Study Design	LOE	Outpatient Definition	N (aTSA, rTSA, HA)	Finding
Basques et al,[12] 2017	Retrospective cohort study	III	Ambulatory surgery	N = 123,347 (both rTSA and aTSA)	Increased rate of 30-d readmission after outpatient TSA for patients aged 85 y or more (OR 34.1, P<.001) compared with patients aged 65–69 y
Biron et al,[20] 2020	Predictive model	IV	<23 h stay	N = 4500 (elective TSA as defined by "arthroplasty, glenohumeral joint")	Longer LOS (≥3 d) for ≥ 70 y of age (P = .001)
Burton et al,[21] 2021	Retrospective cohort study	IV	<23 h stay	N = 17,011 (TSA and HA)	Decreased chance of same-day discharge for age 70.2 ± 10.4 (P<.001)
Carbone et al,[22] 2021	Retrospective cohort study	III	Ambulatory surgery	N = 108,889 (elective aTSA or rTSA)	80–85 age group increased risk of 90-d all-cause readmission in an outpatient setting (OR 3.46; 95% CI, 1.75–6.85; P<.001)
Dunn et al,[23] 2015	Epidemiology study, database analysis	IV	-	N = 2004 inpatient (primary unilateral TSA)	Advanced age (≥80 y vs < 60 y) correlated with increased LOS (OR 2.13; 95% CI, 1.11–4.07; P = .011)

Author, year	Study design	LOE	Outpatient setting	N	Findings
Matsen et al,[31] 2015	Population-based study	III	—	N = 17,311 inpatient ("Primary shoulder Arthroplasty")	66–74 (LOS [multiplicative change:1.04], 90 d readmission [OR:1.69], risk of revision [HR:0.34] $P<.001$ for all); 75–84 (LOS [multiplicative change:1.17], 90 d readmission [OR:3.03], risk of revision [HR:0.19] $P<.001$ for all); >84 (LOS [multiplicative change:1.38], 90 d readmission [OR:3.58], risk of revision [HR:0.07] $P<.001$ for all)
Waterman et al,[27] 2015	Retrospective cohort	III	<23 h stay	N = 2004 (primary unilateral TSA, aTSA, and rTSA)	Age is an independent predictor of mortality and a 2-fold increase for every decade of life (OR 1.19; 95% CI, 1.06–1.33])
Willenbring et al,[28] 2021	Retrospective cohort study	III	Ambulatory surgery	N = 145 (aTSA or rTSA in patients ≥65 y from a single surgeon)	1-y increase in age increased the odds of a surgical complication occurring (OR 1.14, $P = .21$)

Abbreviations: aTSA, anatomic total shoulder arthroplasty; HA, hemiarthroplasty; HR, hazard ratio; LOE, level of evidence; LOS, length of stay; OR, odds ratio; rTSA, reverse total shoulder arthroplasty; TSA, total shoulder arthroplasty.

inconclusive in the literature. In a cross-sectional database study with multivariate analysis of 40,869 patients who underwent elective TSA in either an outpatient (<23 hour stay) or inpatient setting, Menendez and colleagues found that obesity was associated with an increased LOS after aTSA (OR 1.12; 95% CI, 1.02–6.23; $P < .023$) but not rTSA (OR 1.05; 95% CI, 0.88–1.25; $P < .603$).[25] This may be due to an extended LOS being defined as 75th percentile for each cohort or 3 days for aTSA and 4 days for rTSA.[25] Furthermore, in a retrospective review of 1120 unspecified total joint operations (inclusive of TSA, THA, and TKA) performed by a single surgeon, Meneghini and colleagues[24] found lower BMI to be associated with earlier discharge (31.3 vs 32.8 kg/m^2; $t = 3.14$, $P = .002$) (ambulatory surgery). Conversely, in a retrospective review of a single institution shoulder arthroplasty registry and the American College of Surgeons National Surgical Quality Improvement Program (ACS-NSQIP), Steinhaus and colleagues[26] found increased BMI to be associated with likelihood for same-day discharge (OR 1.03, $P = .02$) (<23 hour stay). In addition, Waterman and colleagues[27] did not find obesity to be associated with surgical complications. Given the uncertainty of these findings and relatively weak associations that have been identified, the relationship between BMI and adverse events after TSA may be more nuanced; prior studies in the hip and knee literature have supported the "obesity paradox," whereby obesity has been shown to be protective against adverse medical complications after surgery in a bimodal effect distribution, with the lowest complication rate occurring between a BMI of 35 and 40.[33] The rarity of studies directly comparing BMI as an independent of predictor for (re)admissions, surgical complications, or increased LOS between inpatient and outpatient TSA and their inconclusive findings demonstrates a need for further investigation (Table 2).

Sex

In current studies, outpatient TSA patients are more likely to be male.[10,11] In our review of the literature, several articles supporting a link between sex and LOS in TSA patients were identified. Dunn and colleagues[23] conducted an analysis of patients that underwent primary TSA between 2005 and 2011 in the ACS-NSQIP database and found male sex to be associated with a shorter LOS (OR 0.44; 95% CI, 0.29–0.66; $P < .0001$). Also, in a separate database study of patients undergoing an elective TSA in the ACS-NSQIP between 2011 and 2016, Biron and

colleagues[20] found female sex to be associated with an LOS greater than 1 day (OR 2.67; 95% CI, 2.40–2.96; $P<.0001$). The association between sex and LOS has been confirmed by other studies in TSA and unspecified total joint arthroplasty (TJA) patients.[24,25,31] This discrepancy may be attributable to differing levels of support at home, as Ohwaki and colleagues[34] found marital status found to increase likelihood of early discharge for males but not females in stroke patients. In light of these findings in the literature, social support of patients should be checked, and patients who cannot be discharged to an available caregiver may be more likely to benefit from inpatient TSA. Preoperatively, surgeons should assess patient's support systems to determine whether a caretaker will be available on discharge before recommending outpatient TSA (Table 3).

Comorbidities

An array of medical comorbidities has significance when indicating for outpatient or inpatient care after TSA, namely, heart failure, pulmonary embolism, respiratory failure, diabetes, chronic renal disease, anemia, liver disease, hypothyroidism, and cognitive impairment.[10,11,19,20,23,25–27] No ideal studies directly assessing medical comorbidities as independent predictors for (re)admissions, surgical complications, or increased LOS between inpatient and outpatient TSA were found.

Cardiovascular and Pulmonary Comorbidities

Outpatient TSA patients tend to have fewer cardiovascular comorbidities, but no significant differences in pulmonary comorbidities.[11] However, they have both been identified as predicting patient outcomes and LOS. Cardiovascular comorbidities have been identified as independent risk factors for major morbidity or mortality, decreased odds of same-day discharge, and increased LOS following TSA. Anthony and colleagues[19] identified congestive heart failure (CHF) as an independent predictor for major morbidity within 30 days of surgery (OR 12; 95% CI, 1–106). Waterman and colleagues[27] found a history of CHF or myocardial infarction (MI) to be a significant independent predictor of mortality in TSA patients within 30 days of surgery (OR 62.2; 95% CI, 6.25–619 $P = .0004$). Further, Biron and colleagues[20] found CHF to be a risk factor for increased LOS after TSA (OR 2.92; 95% CI, 1.34–6.37 $P = .0001$), confirming the findings of Menendez and colleagues.[20,25] Waterman and colleagues[27] found that a history of chronic obstructive pulmonary disease (COPD) and

Table 2
Summary of literature evaluating the influence of patient body mass index on eligibility for outpatient total shoulder arthroplasty

Author et al (Year)	Study Design	LOE	Outpatient Definition	N (aTSA, rTSA, HA)	Findings
Meneghini et al, 2021	Retrospective case series	III	Ambulatory surgery	N = 1120 (unspecified total joint arthroplasty)	Lower BMI is associated with a higher likelihood of early discharge (31.3 vs 32.8 kg/m², t = 3.14, P=.002)
Menendez et al,[25] 2015	Cross-sectional database analysis	III	<23 h stay	N = 25,556 (TSA), N = 15,313 (rTSA)	Higher BMI in aTSA patients was associated with extended LOS (OR 1.12; 95% CI, 1.02–6.23; P<.023) but not in rTSA patients (OR 1.05; 95% CI, 0.88–1.25; P<.603)
Waterman et al,[27] 2015	Retrospective cohort	III	<23 h stay	N = 2004 (primary unilateral TSA, aTSA and rTSA)	After controlling for other variables, obesity was not associated with any specified complication.
Steinhaus et al,[26] 2020	Retrospective review	III	<23 h stay	N = 25,556 (aTSA), N = 15,313 (rTSA)	Higher BMI is associated with a higher likelihood for same-day discharge (OR 1.03, P = .02)

Abbreviations: aTSA, anatomic total shoulder arthroplasty; BMI, body mass index; HA, hemiarthroplasty; LOE, level of evidence; LOS, length of stay; OR, odds ratio; rTSA, reverse total shoulder arthroplasty; TSA, total shoulder arthroplasty.

Table 3
Summary of literature evaluating the influence of patient sex on eligibility for outpatient total shoulder arthroplasty

Author et al (Year)	Study Design	LOE	Outpatient Definition	N (aTSA, rTSA, HA)	Findings
Biron et al,[20] 2020	Predictive model	IV	<23 h stay	N = 4500 (elective TSA as defined by "arthroplasty, glenohumeral joint")	Female sex is associated with an LOS over 1 day (OR 2.66; 95% CI, 2.40–2.96; $P<.0001$).
Dunn et al,[23] 2015	Epidemiology study, database analysis	IV	-	N = 2004 (primary unilateral TSA)	Men typically require a shorter LOS (OR 0.44; 95% CI, 0.29–0.66; $P<.0001$).
Matsen et al,[31] 2015	Population-based study	III	-	N = 17,311 ("Primary shoulder Arthroplasty")	Women are associated with an increased LOS (LOS [multiplicative change:0.86]; $P < .001$)
Meneghini et al, 2021	Retrospective case series	III	Ambulatory surgery	N = 1120 (total joint arthroplasty)	Early discharge was more common in men (34.5% vs 22.4%; $P<.0001$)
Menendez et al,[25] 2015	Cross-sectional database analysis	III	<23 h stay	N = 25,556 (aTSA), N = 15,313 (rTSA)	Female gender was an independent predictor of extended LOS in aTSA (OR 2.14; 95% CI, 1.99–2.31; $P<.001$) and rTSA (OR 1.26; 95% CI, 1.10–1.45; $P=.001$)

Abbreviations: aTSA, anatomic total shoulder arthroplasty; BMI, body mass index; CI, confidence interval; HA, hemiarthroplasty; LOE, level of evidence; LOS, length of stay; OR, odds ratio; rTSA, reverse total shoulder arthroplasty; TSA, total shoulder arthroplasty.

peripheral vascular disease were predictive of minor systemic postoperative complications (ie, urinary tract infection, deep venous thrombosis, pneumonia, and renal insufficiency) (OR 6.25; 95% CI, 1.24–31.4; $P = .026$ and OR 3.30; 95% CI, 1.36–8.00; $P = .0085$, respectively). Also, Waterman and colleagues[27] identified COPD as an independent predictor of extended LOS after both aTSA (OR 1.60; 95% CI, 1.45–1.75; $P<.001$) and rTSA (OR 1.54, ; 95% CI, 1.34–1.76; $P<.001$). Considering this evidence from the literature,[35] patients with CHF may be poor candidates for outpatient TSA unless designated as "low" or "low-moderate" risk by a cardiology consult due to the risk of decompensation. The authors also support that a history of MI should also be weighed in the decision process but note that additional research should be done to identify if the timing of the MI impacts the patient risk of mortality and morbidity. In addition, a history of peripheral vascular disease and COPD may be relative contraindications to outpatient TSA, although further research is necessary (Table 4).

Diabetes Mellitus and Renal Comorbidities

Diabetes mellitus (DM), chronic renal disease, and dialysis status have been associated with increased (re)admission and complication rates after TSA and therefore warrant consideration when considering outpatient TSA.[11,23,27,36] Biron and colleagues[20] found DM to be associated with increased LOS following TSA (OR 1.37; 95% CI, 1.20–1.56; $P<.001$), whereas Dunn and colleagues[23] found this to be the case for aTSA (OR 1.40; 95% CI, 1.28–1.52; $P<.001$) but not rTSA on multivariate analysis. Further, Carbone and colleagues[22] found DM to be associated with an increased risk of (re)admission (OR 2.27; 95% CI, 1.42–3.61; $P<.001$) as confirmed by a more recent study by Duey and colleagues.[37] The negative effects of hyperglycemia create potential for more complicated and longer hospital stays, and previous evidence assessing the relationship between postoperative blood glucose levels and periprosthetic joint infection identified a blood glucose cutoff of 137 mg/dL.[38]

Regarding renal comorbidities, dialysis status was associated with increased LOS following TSA (OR 3.62; 95% CI, 1.74–7.51; $P = .023$).[20] Further, Dunn and colleagues[23] found renal insufficiency to be associated with increased LOS after TSA (OR 11.35; 95% CI, 1.68–76.49; $P = .013$), and Menendez and colleagues[25] further demonstrated renal failure to be an independent predictor of extended LOS in aTSA (OR 1.27; 95% CI, 1.08–1.49; $P = .005$) and rTSA (OR

1.65; 95% CI, 1.33–2.05; $P<.001$). Waterman and colleagues[27] concluded renal insufficiency is an independent predictor of mortality and minor systemic complication after TSA (OR 24.2; 95% CI, 1.01–576; $P = .049$). Although renal failure may not preclude a patient from TSA, it may warrant admission after surgery to monitor the return of baseline renal function before discharge home.

Considering this evidence from the literature, renal insufficiency supports admission; however, a hard cutoff has not been identified for kidney function. Poorly-controlled DM requiring close monitoring also supports admission, especially if steroids are given as part of the postoperative pain regimen. A hemoglobin A1c (HgbA1c) of less than 8%[39] is generally accepted as appropriate for elective TSA and a higher HgbA1c may warrant delaying elective TSA until the blood glucose level is better controlled (Table 5).

Medications

Medications, both preoperative and postoperative, warrant consideration in decision-making for outpatient shoulder arthroplasty. Steroids and opioid medications are of particular importance. Using the ACS-NSQIP database, Ling and colleagues[40] studied 1293 TSA on chronic steroids compared with 25,376 TSAs controls and found that preoperative steroid use was independently associated with greater odds of readmission (OR 1.36; 95% CI, 1.04–1.79, $P = .027$), septic shock, urinary tract infection, MI, ventilator requirement greater than 48 hours, non-home discharge, and mortality. Consistent with this finding, Anthony and colleagues[19] found steroid use to be an independent risk factor of postoperative complications in 1922 TSAs (OR, 3; 95% CI, 2–6), as well as an independent risk factor for bleeding necessitating transfusion (OR, 3; 95% CI, 1–6). Waterman and colleagues[27] reported steroid use to be associated with the development of minor systemic complications after controlling for other variables following 2004 TSAs (OR, 3.58, 95% CI, 1.42–9.06). In light of these findings, surgeons should closely monitor patients on steroids and consider postoperative admission for closer monitoring.

In addition, opioids in particular have been extensively reported on in the literature, both as a risk factor for adverse events and lower reported postoperative outcomes.[41–44] Steinhaus and colleagues[26] in their review of 2314 TSAs found a history of narcotic pain medication use to be associated with lower suitability for

Table 4
Summary of literature evaluating the influence of cardiopulmonary comorbidities on eligibility for outpatient total shoulder arthroplasty

Author et al (Year)	Study Design	LOE	Outpatient Definition	N (aTSA, rTSA, HA)	Findings
Anthony et al,[19] 2014	Retrospective cohort	III	-	N = 1922 (TSA)	CHF is an independent predictor for major morbidity or mortality (OR 12; 95% CI, 1–106)
Biron et al,[20] 2020	Predictive model	IV	<23 h stay	N = 4500 (elective TSA as defined by "arthroplasty, glenohumeral joint")	CHF is a risk factor for increased LOS after TSA (OR 2.92; 95% CI, 1.33–6.37 $P = .0001$)
Menendez et al,[25] 2015	Cross-sectional database analysis	III	<23 h stay	N = 25,556 (aTSA), N = 15,313 (rTSA)	CHF was an independent predictor of extended LOS in rTSA (OR 1.89; 95% CI, 1.50–2.37; $P<.001$) and aTSA (OR 2.25; 95% CI, 1.83–2.75; $P<.001$). COPD was also an independent predictor of extended LOS in rTSA (OR 1.54; 95% CI, 1.34–1.76; $P<.001$) and aTSA (OR 1.60; 95% CI, 1.45–1.75; $P<.001$)
Waterman et al,[27] 2015	Retrospective cohort	III	<23 h stay	N = 2004 (primary unilateral TSA, aTSA and rTSA)	History of MI or CHF is a significant independent predictor of mortality in TSA patients (OR 62.22; 95% CI 6.25–619.76 $P = .0004$), whereas COPD and peripheral vascular disease predicted minor systemic complication (OR 6.25; 95% CI, 1.24–31.40] $P = .0262$ and OR 3.30; 95% CI, 1.36–8.00 $P = .0085$, respectively).

Abbreviations: aTSA, anatomic total shoulder arthroplasty; CHF, congestive heart failure; CI, confidence interval; COPD, chronic obstructive pulmonary disease; HA, hemiarthroplasty; LOE, level of evidence; LOS, length of stay; MI, myocardial infarction; OR, odds ratio; rTSA, reverse total shoulder arthroplasty; TSA, total shoulder arthroplasty.

Table 5
Summary of literature evaluating the influence of diabetes mellitus and renal disease on eligibility for outpatient total shoulder arthroplasty

Author et al (Year)	Study Design	LOE	Outpatient Definition	N (aTSA, rTSA, HA)	Findings
Biron et al,[20] 2020	Predictive model	IV	<23 h stay	N = 4500 (elective TSA as defined by "arthroplasty, glenohumeral joint")	DM and dialysis are associated with an increased LOS after TSA (OR 1.37; 95% CI, 1.20–1.56; P = .0001) and (OR 3.62; 95% CI, 1.74–7.50; P = .0234), respectively
Carbone et al,[22] 2021	Retrospective cohort study	III	Ambulatory surgery	N = 108,889 (elective aTSA or rTSA)	DM is associated with increased risk of readmission (OR 2.27; 95% CI, 1.42–3.61; P < .001)
Dunn et al,[23] 2015	Epidemiology study, database analysis	IV	–	N = 2004 (primary unilateral TSA)	Renal insufficiency (OR 11.35; 95% CI, 1.68–76.49; P = .0126) significant risk factor for increased LOS.
Menendez et al,[25] 2015	Cross-sectional database analysis	III	<23 h stay	N = 25,556 (aTSA), N = 15,313 (rTSA)	Renal failure was an independent predictor of extended LOS in rTSA (OR 1.65; 95% CI, 1.33–2.05; P < .001) and aTSA (OR 1.27; 95% CI, 1.08–1.49; P = .005). DM was also an independent predictor of extended LOS, but only in aTSA (OR 1.40; 95% CI, 1.28–1.52; P < .001)
Waterman et al,[27] 2015	Retrospective cohort	III	<23 h stay	N = 2004 (primary unilateral TSA, aTSA and rTSA)	Renal insufficiency is an independent predictor of mortality and minor systemic complication in TSA patients. (OR 24.16; 95% CI, 1.01–576.52; P = .0491)

Abbreviations: aTSA, anatomic total shoulder arthroplasty; CI, confidence interval; DM, diabetes mellitus; HA, hemiarthroplasty; LOE, level of evidence; LOS, length of stay; OR, odds ratio; rTSA, reverse total shoulder arthroplasty; TSA, total shoulder arthroplasty.

same-day discharge (OR, 0.66; $P = .008$). When deciding outpatient versus inpatient TSA, it is important to consider the risk for greater pain medication requirements postoperatively and the safety in discharging a patient who may be taking larger doses of medications that put them at risk at home. Although this may become more manageable with evolving multimodal approaches and regional anesthesia,[45,46] surgeons should use caution when considering same-day discharge for opioid-tolerant patients undergoing TSA due to the risk of uncontrolled pain postoperatively.

Smoking

Smoking presents another complicating factor, with higher postoperative complication rates reported in smokers.[47,48] Ahmed and colleagues[11] reviewed six studies on outpatient (<23 hour stay) TSA ($N = 4368$) compared with inpatient TSA ($N = 133,435$) that specifically evaluated smoking and found that outpatient TSA had a higher prevalence of smokers (8.1 vs 5%, $P<.001$), suggesting smoking status may not be a factor surgeons weigh as particularly important when deciding a patient is a candidate for outpatient TSA. However, Carbone and colleagues[22] retrospectively examined 108,889 elective aTSAs and rTSAs and found smoking to be independently associated with greater 90-day all-cause (re)admission in the outpatient setting (OR 2.24, 95% CI 1.05–4.77). This would seem to indicate that surgeons should closely evaluate the lung function of smokers and use periarticular joint injections in patients with borderline lung function before considering outpatient surgery.

Functional Status and Ability to Ambulate Independently

Functional status and ability to ambulate independently are also significant considerations in outpatient shoulder arthroplasty given the heterogeneity in patient living situations, community support, and availability of help at home or rehabilitation centers. Burton and colleagues[21] evaluated 17,011 aTSA and hemiarthroplasties and found a lower rate of same-day discharge in patients with poor preoperative functional status (ie, independent, poor, or unknown) (4.6% vs 1.6%). In addition, the risk of unplanned (re)admission was higher (OR, 2.8, 95% CI 1.93–3.95) and the same-day discharge rate was lower (OR, 0.53, 95% CI 0.43–0.65) in those with poor functional status. This important variable is infrequently discussed and there remains need for further investigation its effects on outpatient

TSA. Given the limitations set postoperatively after TSA, it would seem that poor functional status and inability to safely ambulate, considering the loss of use of one arm during healing, may preclude certain patients from being considered for outpatient surgery.

Social Characteristics

Social circumstances also inevitably influence patient postoperative outcomes. Biron and colleagues[20] found a shorter LOS associated with white race (OR, 0.57, 95% CI 0.49–0.65). Menendez and colleagues[25] found black race to be associated with longer LOS in aTSA (OR, 1.51, 95% CI, 1.28–1.76).

In addition, mental health is a further consideration. Menendez and colleagues[25] also found depression to be associated with longer LOS in both aTSA and rTSA (aTSA OR, 1.58, 95% CI 1.44–1.73; rTSA OR, 1.15, 95% CI 0.98–1.35), though this was not statistically significant for rTSA. This is notable given depression has previously been shown to be an independent predictor of less improvement postoperatively, increased risk of complications, and increased health care utilization following TSA[49–51] (Table 6).

Preoperative Metrics

Preoperative patient assessments such as ASA class and Charlson–Deyo index score have been previously used to communicate the comorbidity risk profile of patient.[19,52] Ahmed and colleagues[11] reported that outpatient (<23 hour stay) shoulder arthroplasty had significantly lower proportions of ASA class 3 patients (35.2% outpatient vs 48.4% inpatient). Similar to Allahabadi and colleagues[10] and Willenbring and colleagues,[28] Anthony and colleagues[19] found ASA class 4 to be an independent predictor of postoperative medical complication (OR 3; 95% CI 1–7). The investigators also demonstrated ASA class 3 versus 1 or 2 to be an independent risk factor for bleeding resulting in blood transfusion in TSA patients (OR 2; 95% CI 1–5). Biron and colleagues[20] and Dunn and colleagues[23] identified on multivariate logistic regression ASA class $\geq$ 3 to be associated with a longer hospital stay (77% risk of longer hospital stay [$\geq$3 days] for ASA $\geq$ 3 vs 50% for ASA $\leq$ 2 and OR 1.86 for risk of hospital stay with ASA $\geq$ 3, respectively). Waterman and colleagues[27] found ASA class $\geq$ 3 to be associated with minor systemic complications (OR 2.04; 95% CI 1.08–3.85). Steinhaus and colleagues[26] reported Charlson–Deyo index score greater than 2 was associated with decreased suitability for same-day discharge (OR 0.51). These studies support

Table 6
Summary of literature evaluating the influence of smoking, medication, functional status, and patient social factors on eligibility for outpatient total shoulder arthroplasty

Author et al (Year)	Study Design	LOE	Outpatient Definition	N (aTSA, rTSA, HA)	Findings
Ahmed et al,[11] 2021	Systematic review/meta-analysis	III	<23 h stay	10 studies; 7637 outpatient and 192,025 inpatient TSA in total; 6 studies in smoking analysis	The outpatient TSA cohort had a higher prevalence of smokers (6 studies, 4368 outpatient/133,435 inpatient TSA: 8.1% vs 5%) ($P < .001$).
Anthony et al,[19] 2014	Therapeutic study	III	-	N = 1922 (TSA)	Steroid use as independent risk factor of complication (OR 3; 95% CI 2–6) and bleeding resulting in transfusion (OR, 3; 95% CI 1–6).
Biron et al,[20] 2020	Machine learning	IV	<23 h stay	N = 4500 elective TSA	Shorter LOS associated with white race (OR 0.57, 95% CI 0.49–0.65; $P < .001$)
Burton et al,[21] 2021	Retrospective cohort	III	<23 h stay	N = 17,011 (aTSA and HA)	Compared with the rate of non-same-day discharge, the rate of same-day discharge was significantly lower for those with poor functional status (4.6% vs 1.6%, $P < .001$); higher risk of unplanned readmission (OR, 2.8, 95% CI 1.93–3.95, $P < .001$); lower chance of same-day discharge (OR, 0.53, 95% CI 0.43–0.65, $P < .001$)

(continued on next page)

Author et al (Year)	Study Design	LOE	Outpatient Definition	N (aTSA, rTSA, HA)	Findings
Carbone et al,[22] 2021	Retrospective cohort study	III	Ambulatory surgery	N = 108,889 (elective aTSA or rTSA)	Multivariate analysis: smoking associated with risk of 90-d all-cause readmission in the outpatient setting performed (OR 2.24, 95% CI 1.05–4.77, P = .037).
Menendez et al,[25] 2015	Cross-sectional database analysis	III	<23 h stay	N = 25,556 aTSA, 15,313 rTSA	Black race associated with longer LOS in aTSA (OR 1.51; 95% CI, 1.28–1.76; P <.001) Depression associated with longer LOS in both rTSA and aTSA, but not statistically significant in rTSA (rTSA OR; 1.15, 95% CI 0.98–1.35, P = .90; aTSA OR, 1.58, 95% CI 1.44–1.73, P < .001)
Steinhaus et al,[26] 2020	Retrospective review of prospectively collected database	IV	<23 h stay	N = 2314 (aTSA, rTSA, HA)	History of narcotic pain medication use associated with lower suitability for same-day discharge (OR, 0.66; P = .008)
Waterman et al,[27] 2015	Retrospective cohort	III	<23 h stay	N = 2004 (primary unilateral TSA, aTSA and rTSA)	Steroid use associated with minor systemic complication and development of minor systemic complications after control for other variables (OR 3.58; 95% CI 1.42–9.06)

Abbreviations: aTSA, anatomic total shoulder arthroplasty; CI, confidence interval; HA, hemiarthroplasty; LOE, level of evidence; LOS, length of stay; OR, odds ratio; rTSA, reverse total shoulder arthroplasty; TSA, total shoulder arthroplasty.

Table 7
Summary of literature evaluating the relationship between comorbidity indices and eligibility for outpatient total shoulder arthroplasty

Author et al (Year)	Study Design	LOE	Outpatient Definition	N (aTSA, rTSA, HA)	Findings
Ahmed et al,[11] 2021	Systematic review/meta-analysis	III	<23 h stay	10 studies; 7637 outpatient and 192,025 inpatient TSA	ASA class ≥ III (3 studies, 599 outpatient/13,162 inpatient): outpatient 35.2% vs inpatient 48.4%, $P<.001$
Allahabadi et al,[10] 2021	Systematic review/meta-analysis	IV	<23 h stay OR ambulatory surgery	26 studies; total N not reported	Patients undergoing outpatient shoulder arthroplasty were more likely to have a lower ASA score relative to those treated inpatient
Anthony et al,[19] 2014	Therapeutic study	III	-	N = 1922 (TSA)	ASA class 4 was an independent predictor of complication (OR 3; 95% CI, 1–7); ASA class 3 vs 1 or 2 independent risk factors for bleeding resulting in transfusion (OR 2; 95% CI, 1–5); ASA class 4 to be an independent predictor of postoperative medical complication (OR 3; 95% CI 1–7)
Biron et al,[20] 2020	Machine learning	IV	<23 h stay	N = 4500 elective shoulder arthroplasties	Multivariate logistic regression identified ASA class ≥ 3 to be associated with a longer hospital stay (≥3 d) (77 vs 50% for ASA ≤ 2)

(continued on next page)

Author et al (Year)	Study Design	LOE	Outpatient Definition	N (aTSA, rTSA, HA)	Findings
Dunn et al,[23] 2015	Epidemiology study, database analysis	IV	-	N = 2004 (primary unilateral TSA)	Multivariable logistic regression analysis identified ASA class $\geq$3 as a significant risk factor for increased LOS (OR, 1.86; P = .0016).
Steinhaus et al,[26] 2020	Retrospective review of prospectively collected database	IV	<23 h stay	N = 2314 (aTSA, rTSA, HA)	Charlson–Deyo index score > 2 associated with decreased suitability for same day discharge (OR 0.51; P = .009)
Waterman et al,[27] 2015	Retrospective cohort	III	<23 h stay	N = 2004 (primary unilateral TSA)	ASA classification $\geq$ 3 associated with minor systemic complications (OR 2.04; 95% CI 1.08–3.85; P = .027)
Willenbring et al,[28] 2021	Retrospective cohort study	III	Ambulatory surgery	145 primary shoulders (98 inpatient and 47 outpatient); all patients aged $\geq$65 y	ASA score $\geq$3 associated with performing surgery as an inpatient (P<.001)

Abbreviations: ASA, American Society of Anesthesiologists; aTSA, anatomic total shoulder arthroplasty; CI, confidence interval; HA, hemiarthroplasty; LOE, level of evidence; LOS, length of stay; OR, odds ratio; TSA, total shoulder arthroplasty; rTSA, reverse total shoulder arthroplasty.

the use of these measures in stratifying preoperative risk. Furthermore, given the risks and significant comorbidities, surgeons might consider setting a cutoff for an ASA ≤ 2 in order to perform outpatient TSA in the ambulatory surgical center setting where no safety net for medical admission is available (Table 7).

Appropriate patient selection is critical as TSA procedures move from hospitals to ambulatory surgery center (ASCs). As most ASCs have limited or no capacity to host overnight stays, surgeons must recognize which of their patients are good candidates for same-day discharge. Consequently, we have summarized the literature on relevant risk factors associated with early complications and LOS in TSA.

Limitations

This systematic review was limited by the methodological weakness of the included articles. No articles were found which directly assessed the influence of prognostic characteristics on the incidence of adverse outcomes following same-day discharge compared with postoperative admission TSA. Moreover, the lack of consistent outpatient definition among studies decreases the ability to compare studies and generalize findings. Consequently, conclusions and recommendations made by the authors were drawn from unoptimized studies. Another limitation is the lack of a standardized outcome. The studies included reported outcomes ranging from risk of increased LOS to increased patient mortality, precluding the advantages of standardized criteria for measuring a risk factors effect.

SUMMARY

As the demand for TSA increases, the outpatient setting can be used to reduce rising costs while maintaining a high level of patient care. During preoperative assessments, patients should be evaluated for risk factors, which might predispose them to extended LOS or an increased risk of immediate postoperative complications, morbidity, and mortality. The literature reviewed herein suggests that patients with a history of CHF should be admitted postoperatively for monitoring unless cleared by a cardiology consult. In addition, patients with impaired ability to ambulate independently should similarly be admitted postoperatively. Further, age 85+ years, renal insufficiency, poorly controlled DM, and a positive smoking status were identified as risk factors with varying levels of significance for increased LOS or early adverse events. Clinicians should consider these risk factors and the

cumulative risk reflected on patients before recommending outpatient TSA. Future research directly comparing outpatient and inpatient TSA regarding risk factors for early complications and admission is warranted to improve the level of evidence and our knowledge of factors precluding outpatient TSA.

CLINICS CARE POINTS

- As the demand for total shoulder arthroplasty (TSA) increases, the outpatient setting can be used to reduce rising costs while maintaining a high level of patient care.
- Because most ASCs have limited or no capacity to host overnight stays, surgeons must recognize which of their patients are good candidates for same-day discharge.
- Consequently, preoperative assessment for outpatient TSA, patients should be evaluated for risk factors which might predispose them to extended length of stay or an increased risk of immediate postoperative complications, morbidity, and mortality.

DISCLOSURE

Mr K.A. Hao has a consultancy agreement with LinkBio Corp. Dr T.J. Brolin is a consultant for Arthrex, Inc and receives royalties from Arthrex, Inc and Elsevier. Dr J.J. King is a consultant for Exactech, Inc and LinkBio Corp. Dr Wright is a consultant and receives royalties from Exactech, Inc. Dr B.S. Schoch receives royalties from Exactech, Innomed, and Responsive Arthroscopy. The other authors, their immediate families, and any research foundations with which they are affiliated have not received any financial payments or other benefits from any commercial entity related to the subject of this article. Institutional Review Board (IRB): Not applicable given the review did not involve experimentation of human or animal subjects, and the data reviewed are public.

SUPPLEMENTARY DATA

Supplementary data related to this article can be found online at https://doi.org/10.1016/j.ocl.2023.12.002.

REFERENCES

1. Farley KX, Wilson JM, Daly CA, et al. The Incidence of Shoulder Arthroplasty: Rise and Future

Projections Compared to Hip and Knee Arthroplasty. JSES Open Access 2019;3(4):244.

2. Virani NA, Williams CD, Clark R, et al. Preparing for the bundled-payment initiative: the cost and clinical outcomes of total shoulder arthroplasty for the surgical treatment of glenohumeral arthritis at an average 4-year follow-up. J Shoulder Elbow Surg 2013;22(12):1601–11.

3. Arshi A, Leong NL, Wang C, et al. Relative Complications and Trends of Outpatient Total Shoulder Arthroplasty. Orthopedics 2018;41(3):e400–9.

4. Brolin TJ, Mulligan RP, Azar FM, et al. Neer Award 2016: Outpatient total shoulder arthroplasty in an ambulatory surgery center is a safe alternative to inpatient total shoulder arthroplasty in a hospital: a matched cohort study. J Shoulder Elb Surg 2017;26(2):204–8.

5. Cimino AM, Hawkins JK, McGwin G, et al. Is outpatient shoulder arthroplasty safe? A systematic review and meta-analysis. J Shoulder Elb Surg 2021; 30(8):1968–76.

6. Seetharam A, Ghosh P, Prado R, et al. Trends in Outpatient Shoulder Arthroplasty during the COVID-19 era: Increased Proportion of Outpatient Cases with Decrease in 90-day Readmissions. J Shoulder Elb Surg 2022. https://doi.org/10.1016/j.jse.2021.12.031.

7. Leroux TS, Zuke WA, Saltzman BM, et al. Safety and patient satisfaction of outpatient shoulder arthroplasty. JSES Open Access 2018;2(1):13–7.

8. Puzzitiello RN, Moverman MA, Pagani NR, et al. Current Status Regarding the Safety of Inpatient Versus Outpatient Total Shoulder Arthroplasty: A Systematic Review. HSS Journal®. 2022;18(3):428–38.

9. Brolin TJ, Cox RM, Zmistowski BM, et al. Surgeons' experience and perceived barriers with outpatient shoulder arthroplasty. J Shoulder Elbow Surg 2018;27(6S):S82–7.

10. Allahabadi S, Cheung EC, Hodax JD, et al. Outpatient Shoulder Arthroplasty-A Systematic Review. J Shoulder Elb Arthroplast 2021;5. 247154922 11028025.

11. Ahmed AF, Hantouly A, Toubasi A, et al. The safety of outpatient total shoulder arthroplasty: a systematic review and meta-analysis. Int Orthop 2021; 45(3):697–710.

12. Basques BA, Erickson BJ, Leroux T, et al. Comparative outcomes of outpatient and inpatient total shoulder arthroplasty: an analysis of the Medicare dataset. Bone Jt J 2017;99-B(7):934–8.

13. Calkins TE, Mosher ZA, Throckmorton TW, et al. Safety and Cost Effectiveness of Outpatient Total Shoulder Arthroplasty: A Systematic Review. J Am Acad Orthop Surg 2022;30(2):e233–41.

14. Erickson BJ, Shishani Y, Jones S, et al. Outpatient versus inpatient anatomic total shoulder arthroplasty: outcomes and complications. JSES Int 2020;4(4):919–22.

15. Huddleston HP, Mehta N, Polce EM, et al. Complication rates and outcomes after outpatient shoulder arthroplasty: a systematic review. JSES Int 2021;5(3):413–23.

16. Kucharik MP, Varady NH, Best MJ, et al. Comparison of outpatient vs. inpatient anatomic total shoulder arthroplasty: a propensity score-matched analysis of 20,035 procedures. JSES Int 2022;6(1):15–20.

17. Nwankwo CD, Dutton P, Merriman JA, et al. Outpatient Total Shoulder Arthroplasty Does Not Increase the 90-Day Risk of Complications Compared With Inpatient Surgery in Prescreened Patients. Orthopedics 2018;41(4):e563–8.

18. O'Donnell EA, Fury MS, Maier SP 2nd, et al. Outpatient Shoulder Arthroplasty Patient Selection, Patient Experience, and Cost Analyses: A Systematic Review. JBJS Rev 2021;9(11). https://doi.org/10.2106/JBJS.RVW.20.00235.

19. Anthony CA, Westermann RW, Gao Y, et al. What Are Risk Factors for 30-day Morbidity and Transfusion in Total Shoulder Arthroplasty? A Review of 1922 Cases. Clin Orthop Relat Res 2015;473(6):2099–105.

20. Biron DR, Sinha I, Kleiner JE, et al. A Novel Machine Learning Model Developed to Assist in Patient Selection for Outpatient Total Shoulder Arthroplasty. J Am Acad Orthop Surg 2020;28(13):e580–5.

21. Burton BN, Finneran JJ, Angerstein A, et al. Demographic and clinical factors associated with same-day discharge and unplanned readmission following shoulder arthroplasty: a retrospective cohort study. Korean J Anesthesiol 2021;74(1):30–7.

22. Carbone A, Vervaecke AJ, Ye IB, et al. Outpatient versus inpatient total shoulder arthroplasty: A cost and outcome comparison in a comorbidity matched analysis. J Orthop 2021;28:126–33.

23. Dunn JC, Lanzi J, Kusnezov N, et al. Predictors of length of stay after elective total shoulder arthroplasty in the United States. J Shoulder Elbow Surg 2015;24(5):754–9.

24. Meneghini RM, Ziemba-Davis M, Ishmael MK, et al. Safe Selection of Outpatient Joint Arthroplasty Patients With Medical Risk Stratification: the "Outpatient Arthroplasty Risk Assessment Score.". J Arthroplasty 2017;32(8):2325–31.

25. Menendez ME, Baker DK, Fryberger CT, et al. Predictors of extended length of stay after elective shoulder arthroplasty. J Shoulder Elbow Surg 2015;24(10):1527–33.

26. Steinhaus ME, Liu JN, Gowd AK, et al. The Feasibility of Outpatient Shoulder Arthroplasty: Risk Stratification and Predictive Probability Modeling. Orthopedics 2021;44(2):e215–22.

27. Waterman BR, Dunn JC, Bader J, et al. Thirty-day morbidity and mortality after elective total shoulder arthroplasty: patient-based and surgical risk factors. J Shoulder Elbow Surg 2015;24(1):24–30.

28. Willenbring TJ, DeVos MJ, Kozemchak AM, et al. Is outpatient shoulder arthroplasty safe in patients aged ≥65 years? A comparison of readmissions and complications in inpatient and outpatient settings. J Shoulder Elb Surg 2021;30(10):2306–11.

29. Moher D, Liberati A, Tetzlaff J, et al, The PRISMA Group. Preferred Reporting Items for Systematic Reviews and Meta-Analyses: The PRISMA Statement. PLoS Med 2009;6(7):e1000097.

30. Ambulatory Surgery - an overview | ScienceDirect Topics. Available at: https://www.sciencedirect.com/topics/medicine-and-dentistry/ambulatory-surgery. Accessed August 21, 2023

31. Matsen FA, Li N, Gao H, et al. Factors Affecting Length of Stay, Readmission, and Revision After Shoulder Arthroplasty: A Population-Based Study. J Bone Joint Surg Am 2015;97(15):1255–63.

32. Mehta N, Bohl DD, Cohn MR, et al. Trends in outpatient versus inpatient total shoulder arthroplasty over time. JSES Int 2022;6(7):7–14.

33. Smith EL, Shahien AA, Chung M, et al. The Obesity Paradox: Body Mass Index Complication Rates Vary by Gender and Age Among Primary Total Hip Arthroplasty Patients. J Arthroplasty 2020;35(9):2658–65.

34. Ohwaki K, Hashimoto H, Sato M, et al. Gender and family composition related to discharge destination and length of hospital stay after acute stroke. Tohoku J Exp Med 2005;207(4):325–32.

35. Imam N, Sudah SY, Manzi JE, et al. Perioperative risk stratification tools for shoulder arthroplasty: a systematic review. J Shoulder Elbow Surg 2023;32(6):e293–304.

36. King JJ, Patrick MR, Struk AM, et al. Perioperative Factors Affecting the Length of Hospitalization After Shoulder Arthroplasty. J Am Acad Orthop Surg Glob Res Rev 2017;1(6):e026.

37. Duey AH, White CA, Levy KH, et al. Diabetes increases risk for readmission and infection after shoulder arthroplasty: A national readmissions study of 113,713 patients. J Orthop 2023;38:25–9.

38. Kheir MM, Tan TL, Kheir M, et al. Postoperative Blood Glucose Levels Predict Infection After Total Joint Arthroplasty. J Bone Jt Surg 2018;100(16):1423–31.

39. Cancienne JM, Brockmeier SF, Werner BC. Association of Perioperative Glycemic Control With Deep Postoperative Infection After Shoulder Arthroplasty in Patients With Diabetes. JAAOS - J Am Acad Orthop Surg. 2018;26(11):e238.

40. Ling K, Kim M, Nazemi A, et al. Chronic steroid use and readmission following total shoulder arthroplasty. JSES Int 2022;6(5):775–80.

41. Jones CA, Throckmorton TW, Murphy J, et al. Opioid-sparing pain management protocol after shoulder arthroplasty results in less opioid consumption and higher satisfaction: a prospective, randomized controlled trial. J Shoulder Elbow Surg 2022;31(10):2057–65.

42. Baessler A, Smith PJ, Brolin TJ, et al. Preoperative opioid usage predicts markedly inferior outcomes 2 years after reverse total shoulder arthroplasty. J Shoulder Elbow Surg 2022;31(3):608–15.

43. Berglund DD, Rosas S, Kurowicki J, et al. Preoperative Opioid Use Among Patients Undergoing Shoulder Arthroplasty Predicts Prolonged Postoperative Opioid Use. J Am Acad Orthop Surg 2018;27(15):e691–5.

44. Martusiewicz A, Khan AZ, Chamberlain AM, et al. Outpatient narcotic consumption following total shoulder arthroplasty. JSES Int 2020;4(1):100–4.

45. Sethi PM, Mandava NK, Liddy N, et al. Narcotic requirements after shoulder arthroplasty are low using a multimodal approach to pain. JSES Int 2021;5(4):722–8.

46. Weir TB, Simpson N, Aneizi A, et al. Single-shot liposomal bupivacaine interscalene block versus continuous interscalene catheter in total shoulder arthroplasty: Opioid administration, pain scores, and complications. J Orthop 2020;22:261–7.

47. Hatta T, Werthel JD, Wagner ER, et al. Effect of smoking on complications following primary shoulder arthroplasty. J Shoulder Elbow Surg 2017;26(1):1–6.

48. Althoff AD, Reeves RA, Traven SA, et al. Smoking is associated with increased surgical complications following total shoulder arthroplasty: an analysis of 14,465 patients. J Shoulder Elbow Surg 2020;29(3):491–6.

49. Werner BC, Wong AC, Chang B, et al. Depression and Patient-Reported Outcomes Following Total Shoulder Arthroplasty. J Bone Jt Surg 2017;99(8):688–95.

50. Lunati MP, Wilson JM, Farley KX, et al. Preoperative depression is a risk factor for complication and increased health care utilization following total shoulder arthroplasty. J Shoulder Elbow Surg 2021;30(1):89–96.

51. Mollon B, Mahure SA, Ding DY, et al. The influence of a history of clinical depression on peri-operative outcomes in elective total shoulder arthroplasty: a ten-year national analysis. Bone Jt J 2016;98-B(6):818–24.

52. Westermann RW, Anthony CA, Duchman KR, et al. Incidence, Causes and Predictors of 30-Day Readmission After Shoulder Arthroplasty. Iowa Orthop J 2016;36:70–4.

Foot and Ankle

Considerations Regarding Vitamin D in Foot and Ankle Treatment and Surgery

James D. Michelson, MD

KEYWORDS

- Vitamin D • Hypovitaminosis D • Fracture healing • Foot and ankle surgery

KEY POINTS

- Hypovitaminosis D is very common in the foot and ankle (F&A) patient population.
- Supplementation of vitamin D (200IU/d) and calcium (1gm/d) is safe and can promote healing in fractures and fusion.
- Patients with fragility fractures (low-energy injuries that should not cause fracture) should be referred for assessment for osteoporosis.
- Although there is a high prevalence of hypovitaminosis D among diabetic patients, patients with osteochondritis dissecans, and bone marrow edema syndrome, no cause-and-effect relationship has been established.

ROLE OF VITAMIN D IN CALCIUM METABOLISM

Vitamin D plays a critical and central role in calcium metabolism. In concert with parathyroid hormone (PTH), it acts to maintain serum calcium levels. Although one can obtain vitamin D from routine dietary sources, this tends to be a minor contributor, accounting for between 10% and 20% of normal vitamin D requirements.[1–4] Exposure to sunlight provides the bulk of vitamin D synthesis, where UVB radiation acts to form vitamin D3.[2] Dietary sources from plant and fungal sources form a different form of vitamin D, termed D2, whereas dietary sources from meat and fish form D3.[2,4] This is important, as D3 is much more readily converted in the liver to 25-hydroxy vitamin D. Consequently, oral supplementation with the D3 form is more effective in restoring serum vitamin D levels then supplementing with D2.[5,6] The circulating levels of 1-hydroxy D are what is typically measured clinically, as it has a half-life of 3 weeks.[2] The mono-hydroxylate vitamin D is then converted in the kidney to either 1,25-dihydroxy D, which is the

active form of vitamin D, or 24,25-dihydroxy D, which is the inactive form of vitamin D; 1,25-dihydroxy D has a half-life of only 4 hours, so it is not typically measured in the clinical setting.[2]

Vitamin D has several sites of action (Fig. 1). It increases intestinal absorption of calcium in the GI tract, promotes mineralization in bones, and increases calcium and phosphorus absorption in the kidney.[7] Serum calcium levels are critical to normal functioning of virtually all cellular metabolism, so maintaining it with in a tight range is imperative. Ninety-nine percent of bodily calcium is contained in the bones and teeth, with the interplay between vitamin D and PTH providing the primary source of regulating the release of calcium from, or its deposition into, bone.[3] Consequently, calcium and vitamin D deficiency leads to bone loss as the bone calcium stores are harvested to maintain serum calcium levels.[4] Low calcium triggers an increase in PTH levels, which subsequently causes an increase in kidney conversion to the active 1,25-dihydroxy D form, which increases calcium resorption and increases phosphate excretion. In contrast, high serum calcium levels

Orthopaedic Surgery, Department of Orthopaedics and Rehabilitation, Larner College of Medicine, University of Vermont, Stafford Hall 418, 95 Carrigan Drive, Burlington, VT 05401, USA
E-mail address: James.michelson@uvm.edu

Orthop Clin N Am 55 (2024) 383–392
https://doi.org/10.1016/j.ocl.2024.01.002
0030-5898/24/© 2024 Elsevier Inc. All rights reserved.

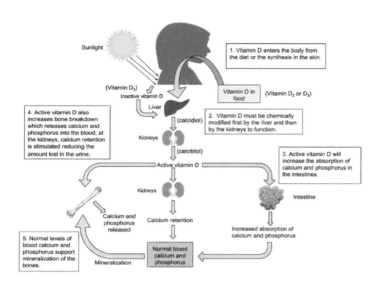

induce increased calcitonin release from the thyroid, which inhibits osteoclast activity, decreases calcium resorption in the kidney, and decreases calcium absorption in the GI tract.

Vitamin D also has direct actions on osteogenesis through binding to the DNA as a transcription factor affecting RANKL receptor synthesis and influencing the production of osteocalcin and osteopontin.[7] The extent of these actions is influenced by the presence of estrogen as well as PTH. Vitamin D and PTH also bind to the RANKL receptor to cause increase bone resorption, which increases serum calcium. Finally, vitamin D provides negative feedback to its own production by prompting metabolization of 25-hydroxy vitamin D and 1,25-dihydroxy vitamin D.

There is some debate in the literature regarding the physiologically appropriate levels needed for normal calcium homeostasis in humans. The Endocrine Society guidelines published in 2011[8] defined more than 30 ng/mL serum vitamin D as adequate, between 20 and 30 ng/mL as insufficiency and less than 20 ng/mL as deficiency. This is the most common guideline cited in the literature. The rationale for choosing these cutoffs for defining normal and abnormal levels of vitamin D have to do with the physiology of low vitamin D levels. Vitamin D levels less than 20 ng/mL are associated with increased expression of PTH, indicating the need for a higher level of vitamin D to maintain serum calcium. In addition, serum vitamin D below 30 ng/mL are associated with mineralization defects in bone,[3] indicating that levels above this are needed to avoid osteomalacia.

In contrast, the Institute of Medicine[5] suggested that the appropriate levels for sufficiency should be 50 ng/mL and for deficiency being less than 30 ng/mL.

Throughout this review, the author uses the definitions recommended by the Endocrine Society while recognizing that there is some ongoing discussion. To avoid confusion, this review will only use vitamin D measurement units of ng/mL. An alternative measurement is mmole/liter,[9] which is used in many studies. All such measurements will be reported here as ng/mL, using the conversion factors 75 mmol/L = 30 ng/mL, and 50 mmol/L = 20 ng/mL.

The recommended daily requirement for vitamin D by the Endocrine Society is 600 IU/day in patients less than 70 year old, increasing to 800 IU/day in those more than 70.[8] However, they do note that if the goal is to achieve a 30 ng/mL serum level, 1500 IU to 2000 IU/day is needed. It has also been recommended that patients at risk for hypovitaminosis D (inadequate sunlight, certain medications, and so forth) should consider taking between 800 IU and 1000 IU daily.[1,4]

EPIDEMIOLOGY OF HYPOVITAMINOSIS D

Despite widespread recognition of the need to maintain adequate vitamin D levels, the prevalence of hypovitaminosis D is "endemic."[3] In the foot and ankle (F&A) population, up to 75% of unselected patients have been found with hypovitaminosis D.[10–14] In a study of 98 ankle fracture surgery patients in a mid-Atlantic level 1 trauma center (40° N Latitude), 39% of the patients had vitamin D levels that were insufficient and another 36% had deficient vitamin D levels.[10] Among patients having elective foot surgery, hypovitaminosis D was seen in 34%, which was lower than the 88% in the orthopedic trauma group.[13] In a prospective study of ankle and hindfoot fusions in New England (44° N Latitude), 67% of 81 patients had hypovitaminosis D.[14] These reports mirror those seen from general unselected population surveys, with hypovitaminosis D ranging from 50% at mid-latitude sites to more than 90% at high-latitude sites.[15–18]

There are some risk factors for hypovitaminosis D which are not controversial. Perhaps most notable is living at a more northern latitude,[2,4,5,19] with one study demonstrating a linear relationship between latitude and rate of hypovitaminosis D.[20] One meta-analysis, though, suggested that this relationship was only true for people with white skin and not people of color.[21] Consistent with the concept that people living in northern latitudes get less sun exposure, most studies have shown an increase in hypovitaminosis D in the winter as opposed to the summer,[1,2,17,22–27] although this is not universally found.[28] Darker skin also has a strong association with hypovitaminosis D.[2,5,8,12,19,21,23,29–33] The physiologic basis of this is the increased melanin in their skin blocks the UVB radiation that drives the synthesis of vitamin D. Similarly, sunscreen use, which blocks UVB radiation, reduces the endogenous production of vitamin D in the skin.[4,8]

Obesity, or having undergone bariatric surgery, is also a well-recognized cause of hypovitaminosis D, most likely due to the associated malabsorption syndromes in such patients.[1,2,5,8,9,11,34] This, however, is not always detected.[9,10,35] The influence of age as a risk for low vitamin D is not clear, with many conflicting reports. What does seem to be true is that elderly patients who spend most of their time indoors and do not have supplementation of vitamin D are likely at higher risk.[1,2,5,8] Patients with renal disease or liver disease are also at risk for low vitamin D due to the impaired vitamin conversion in those organs.[1,5,9,34] Sex does not seem to be an independent risk factor other than in postmenopausal females, which is primarily due to estrogen deficiency issues rather than sex. Several classes of medications are known to interfere with vitamin D metabolism or action, including steroids, anti-seizure medications, antiretroviral medications, cholestyramine, rifampin, and antifungal medications.[1,9,34] Granulomatous diseases such as sarcoidosis or tuberculosis are also associated with higher rates of hypovitaminosis D.[34] Smoking has not been shown to be a risk factor for low vitamin D.

CONSEQUENCES OF HYPOVITAMINOSIS D

The consequences of hypovitaminosis D can be predicted based on its physiology, which is targeted to maintain serum calcium by improving absorption of calcium and decreasing excretion of calcium. In the face of low vitamin D, PTH increases to maintain serum calcium by liberation of calcium in the bones and increasing calcium resorption in the kidney at the expense of increasing phosphate excretion.[4,8] This results in decreased bone mineral density (BMD) due to decreased mineralization of osteoid and increased absorption of bone from osteoclast activation by PTH.[4,8] In a study of patients with femoral neck fractures, 99% had low vitamin D and exhibited impaired mineralization of osteoid in the femoral neck along with above normal PTH levels compared with age-matched controls.[36] In children, low vitamin D leads to rickets due to the mineralization defect in osteoid, whereas in adults this manifests as osteomalacia.[8,37]

There are many other hypothesized correlations with low vitamin D that are, as yet, unproven. Muscle weakness, which leads to increased falls and fractures in the elderly, is accepted as a consequence of hypovitaminosis D.[1,2,8]

VITAMIN D SUPPLEMENTATION

The role of vitamin D supplementation is surprisingly controversial. From an academic standpoint, rigorous studies conclusively showing the benefit of supplementation are few and far between. The reason for this is that many studies include a majority of patients with normal vitamin D levels, who would not be expected to benefit from supplemental vitamin D. Vitamin D can be thought of as a threshold nutrient.[38] Increasing amounts of such a nutrient improve function up to a certain threshold, which in the case of vitamin D would be set at 30 ng/mL by most authors. However, above that level, which is the situation in most clinical studies, adding more of the nutrient will not have any further benefit.

Although it has been stated that there is not much support for universal vitamin D supplementation,[6] several studies of orthopedic patients have found such a high rate of hypovitaminosis D that routine vitamin D supplementation would be cost-effective.[34,39–41] In a prospective study of 144 orthopedic trauma patients, 97% of whom started with low vitamin D, 100% of patients achieved normal serum vitamin D levels after being placed on 600 IU daily for 6 months. Another prospective study of 81 patients undergoing ankle and hindfoot fusions[14] found that a 2-month regimen of high-dose vitamin D supplementation achieved normal vitamin D levels in only 56% of patients. The cost of supplementation is very low, particularly compared with the potential cost savings of avoiding a small number of nonunions.[34,40] Similarly, the risks of vitamin D toxicity are extremely low, with no complications reported in any of the supplementation studies.[4,18,34,42] The endocrinology guidelines note that up to 10,000 IU D3 daily for 5 months is safe.[4]

OSTEOPENIA AND OSTEOPOROSIS

Osteopenia progressing to osteoporosis, while not directly related to vitamin D metabolism, also impacts the types of fractures and treatment of fractures presenting to the F&A surgeon. Osteoporosis is defined as BMD less than 2.5 SD below the mean young adult levels and is most commonly related to the lack of estrogen in postmenopausal women.[3] In addition to putting patients at increased risk for fragility fractures (low-energy injuries that would not otherwise result in a fracture), such patients have a higher rate of complications after fractures and may take longer to heal.[3]

Although not the primary province of orthopedic surgeons, a general knowledge of the treatment of osteoporosis is important in treating such patients. Vitamin D by itself is not effective in reducing fracture rate.[1,3,43–45] This changes by the addition of calcium to vitamin D supplementation, which is generally reported to reduce the incidence of hip and non-spine fractures.[1,3,8,38,43,44] Although there is one study that compared 99 patients with metatarsal fractures to 28 control patients and found no difference in vitamin D levels, low vitamin D was found in more than 90% of both groups making any conclusion regarding the role of vitamin D problematic.[29]

The initial medications used to treat osteoporosis were of the antiresorptive type. This is represented by bisphosphonates and denosumab (a monoclonal antibody to RANKL). Unfortunately, the bisphosphonates can only be used for 5 years before the rate of atypical fractures become a clinical concern.[38,46] Denosumab does not have this limitation.[38] These medications have been supplanted as first-line drugs by the advent of osteoanabolic medications, exemplified by teriparatide which is human recombinant PTH. These medications have been shown to increase bone ingrowth into implants as well as decreased non-vertebral fractures.[47,48]

VITAMIN D AND HEALING OF FUSIONS AND FRACTURES

Although the physiology of vitamin D and calcium metabolism lends intuitive sense to the concept that vitamin D plays a role in fracture and fusion healing, the data in humans are quite limited. There are several reasons for this, not the least of which is that many of the clinical studies involve populations that have low vitamin D prevalence of less than 10%.[1] Because vitamin D is a threshold nutrient,[38] supplementation of vitamin D in a predominantly normal vitamin D population would not be expected to have any beneficial effects. Another issue is the difficulty in detecting a significant decrease in nonunion rates. In one study of fracture healing and a level 1 trauma center, it was estimated that it would take a study size of 180,000 patients to detect a 5% reduction in nonunion rate.[40] In discussing the results of ankle and hindfoot fusions, it was noted that to detect an increase of nonunion rate due to hypovitaminosis D from 15% to 30% in a high-risk group would require a total of 300 patients in the study, larger than any previous published study.[14]

There have been several animal models that have demonstrated improved callus formation, improved mineralization of callus, improved torsional strength, and accelerated healing in various fracture studies.[5,6,49–52] In an oophorectomy model involving rats, vitamin D supplementation improved histologic healing and mechanical strength.[53]

The clinical evidence in humans is much more mixed. One prospective randomized control trial involving proximal humerus fractures were given vitamin D plus calcium versus placebo for 12 weeks.[54] This resulted in improved callus and BMD at the fracture site compared with controls and improved serum vitamin D from a starting value of 16 to 29 ng/mL. A retrospective study of 47 ankle fusions showed that 100% of the nonunions occurred in patients with low vitamin D,[55] whereas another retrospective study of nonunions versus healed fractures showed that hypovitaminosis D increase the risk of nonunion eightfold.[56] Another retrospective study reported that six patients healed their nonunions after referral to endocrinology and appropriate supplementation.[57] A recent narrative review of the literature expressed the conclusion that the literature supports the concept that hypovitaminosis D increases nonunion rate and, conversely, daily vitamin D plus calcium supplementation improved fracture healing.[2] In contrast, there are many studies and meta-analyses that have found the effect of vitamin D on fracture healing to be inconsistent.[58–61] However, the lack of evidence is not evidence of no role for vitamin D in bone healing, as was noted in the most recent umbrella meta-analysis, "The limitations of our findings are in large part due to the limitation of the evidence available."[58]

EFFECT ON FUNCTIONAL OUTCOMES AFTER FRACTURE

Once the patient with hypovitaminosis D presents with a fracture, the question arises regarding whether they are at increased risk for poor outcomes. With respect to ankle fractures, one study found that low vitamin D impaired activities of daily living scores on the AOFAS ankle outcome score but had no other effects on the clinical outcome.[10] Overall complication rates do not seem to be increased in some studies following fracture surgery,[10,42] whereas one study of tibial fractures found that a high rate of nonunion when vitamin D levels was below 10 ng/mL.[2] Mortality following hip fractures does seem to be increased in patients with vitamin D levels below 20 ng/mL.[2]

INCIDENCE AND HEALING OF STRESS FRACTURES

The role of vitamin D in stress fractures has been examined in both the athletic and military context. Among military recruits, hypovitaminosis D is common, being seen in up to 70% of subjects.[35] The most common site for stress fracture among military recruits was the femoral neck, with F&A stress fractures occurring less commonly. There is no clear relationship between the incidence of F&A stress fractures and vitamin D,[35,62] with one study finding longer recovery from stress fractures when vitamin D levels were below 20 ng/mL.[63] One retrospective study of 124 patients with F&A stress fractures found that 77% of the fractures were of the metatarsals, with hypovitaminosis D noted in 53% of patients.[64] A review of the subject stated that although vitamin D alone does not reduce fracture risk, the addition of calcium supplementation does reduce stress fracture risk.[65]

INSUFFICIENCY (FRAGILITY) FRACTURES

Fragility fractures are defined as fractures that result from low-energy injuries that would not result in a fracture if the patient had normal bones. There is a single prospective case-control study of fragility fractures, 89% of which were of the metatarsals.[66] Unfortunately, 20/55 fracture patients were on steroids compared

with none of the 40 controls, so no conclusions can be drawn relative to vitamin D status. It was noted, however, that the metatarsal stress fracture patients had higher calcaneal pitch and metatarsus adductus compared with controls.

When encountering a stress fracture, it should be treated as sentinel event because there is a high likelihood of subsequent fracture without intervention.[67] As the orthopedist is likely to be the first person involved in the patients care, it is important to proactively identify these injuries and initiate treatment for the underlying skeletal disorder, optimally as part of an integrated fracture liaison service. The assessment of the extent the disorder and estimation of subsequent fracture risk includes obtaining dual-energy X-ray absorptiometry (DEXA) scanning, vertebral fracture assessment radiographically, and detailing of relevant comorbidities. Skeletal BMD deficits should be aggressively treated, typically by an endocrinologist, particularly if the DEXA score is less than -2.5 or if there is a prior hip or spine fracture history, or if the 10-year risk of a hip fracture exceeds 3% and that of a long bone fracture exceeds 20% using the fracture risk assessment (FRAX) tool.[68]

An interesting phenomenon of secondary demineralization after fracture has been observed. After hip fracture, the contralateral hip has a decrease in BMD of up to 5% with spinal BMD decreasing up to 15%.[3] This suggests that there is a need for increased calcium for fracture healing that is mobilized from distant sites. This may be accentuated when patients already have low vitamin D or low calcium intake. As such, vitamin D and calcium supplementation during fracture healing should be considered to prevent systemic bone loss and reduce future fracture risk. Given the different responses that folks have seen to vitamin D supplementation (as noted in the Supplementation section), there are no specific recommendations for supplementation following fracture. The author's own personal recommendation is 2000 IU/day of vitamin D and 1 gm/day calcium.

VITAMIN D IN DIABETES

Hypovitaminosis D is endemic among patients with diabetes, being reported in 79% of diabetic patients in one retrospective study.[69] Although there seems to be an inverse relationship between vitamin D levels and population prevalence of diabetes, there are many confounding variables (obesity, age, comorbidities) that prevent any firm conclusions from being drawn from this association.[25] The observation that vitamin D may be lower in diabetic patients with neuropathy versus those without neuropathy[69] does not imply any cause-and-effect relationship for the same reason. Interestingly', vitamin D levels do not seem to be different between diabetic patients with or without Charcot neuroarthropathy.[69,70] Because it was observed that Charcot neuroarthropathy was associated with decreased BMD,[70] treatment directed at restoring BMD in such patients has been tested. A recent prospective randomized trial[71] compared the administration of teriparatide with vitamin D and calcium versus placebo with vitamin D and calcium for healing of Charcot foot fractures. They reported no improvement in clinical or radiographic healing or reduction in bone turnover markers, indicating that recombinant PTH does not enhance Charcot fracture resolution.

OSTEOCHONDRITIS DISSECANS

There have been several retrospective studies suggesting that hypovitaminosis D plays a role in the etiology of osteochondritis dissecans. In 40 juveniles with OCD, 70% of which were in the F&A, 45% of patients exhibited hypovitaminosis D.[25] In a study that matched patients with idiopathic osteochondritis dissecans (OCD) versus traumatic OCD, 75% of all patients had low vitamin D without a difference between the two groups.[22] In contrast, in a retrospective study of 80 patients with OCD (61% talus, 30% femoral condyle) were age-matched against controls,[72] vitamin D levels were significantly lower in the OCD group than the control group (10 ng/mL vs 26 ng/mL). Using multivariate progression in a retrospective study of 46 patients with talar OCD and 40 controls, hypovitaminosis D conveyed a 45% increased risk of having an OCD.

BONE MARROW EDEMA SYNDROME

Bone marrow edema syndrome (BMES) is defined by the presence of bone pain without associated fractures or identifiable etiology other than bone marrow edema visualized on MRI, with increased signal on T2 and decreased signal on T1 imaging. Other terminology for this syndrome includes transient osteoporosis, transient bone marrow edema, and patients identified as having "severe nonspecific musculoskeletal pain." Although these imaging findings can be secondary to trauma, inflammatory conditions, malignancy, infection, and so forth, in the absence of any such underlying cause, primary BMES is the diagnosis assigned. The most common site of the BMES is the femoral head, with F&A sites being second most common (roughly 30% of cases).[73,74]

It has been hypothesized that hypovitaminosis D may be a cause of this condition.[73,74] The rationale for this being that vitamin D causes decrease in mineralization which leads to abnormal bone structure and symptoms. There have been three retrospective case series published regarding the association of vitamin D and BMES. In a retrospective study of 65 patients, the peak age for symptoms was found to be adolescence and in those between 50 and 70 years of age.[74] BMES was in the F&A in 55% and hypovitaminosis D detected in 91% of patients. In two other retrospective case series limited to F&A BMES involving 31 patients[75] and 10 patients,[76] hypovitaminosis D was found in 84% and 90% of patients, respectively.

An example of such a patient is shown in **Fig. 2**. This patient had a 1-year history of idiopathic pain in his heel that was completely limiting his ability to walk. He has been immobilized multiple times

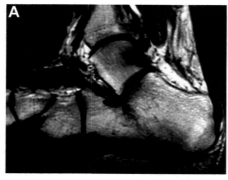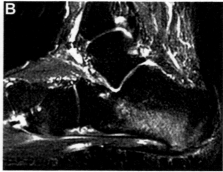

Fig. 2. MRI images of patient with clinical symptoms consistent with bone marrow edema syndrome (BMES). (A) T1-weighted images that show reduced signal in the inferior body of the calcaneus. (B) T2-weighted images showing markedly increased signal in the calcaneus corresponding to both the decreased T1 signal area and the location of tenderness.

as well as placed non-weight-bearing, none of which helped his pain. His vitamin D levels were measured and found to be 18 ng/mL. He was started on high-dose vitamin D replacement (50,000 IU 3 times a week × 2 months). Within 1 week after starting his vitamin D supplementation, his pain significantly lessened, and within 1 month was completely resolved.

SUMMARY

Although vitamin D has a complex role in calcium homeostasis and bone metabolism, there continues to be uncertainty as to the degree of impact that vitamin D has on the incidence of fractures in the F&A or the healing of F&A fractures or fusions. Notwithstanding this, it is known that there is a very large therapeutic window for the use of vitamin D, which is very inexpensive and does not require ongoing monitoring. The academic arguments regarding the precise level of vitamin D that is required do not address the practical needs of most patients. The literature would support the uniform use of vitamin D supplementation, generally about 2000 IU/day, in conjunction with calcium (1 g/day) to maintain adequate levels of vitamin D in most, if not all, patients. Given the lack of toxicity of such a dose as well as the low cost, this seems a reasonable, practical way to ensure adequate vitamin D levels to promote optimal bone health and healing. In patients who have sustained fractures, the phenomenon of secondary demineralization (where nonfracture bones lose calcium to provide calcium for fracture healing) should be prevented by vitamin D and calcium supplementation.

Although orthopedic F&A surgeons are not expected to be the experts in managing derangements of calcium metabolism that result in osteoporosis or osteomalacia, it is important for us to maintain vigilance because we frequently are the first provider to detect the harbingers of such disorders by the presence of stress fractures or fragility fractures. In these circumstances, recognition of the underlying potential problem should trigger referral to the appropriate specialist for ongoing assessment and treatment.

Currently, there is circumstantial evidence suggesting a role of hypovitaminosis D in BMES and possibly osteochondritis dissecans. There should be a low threshold for assessing vitamin D levels in such patients to make sure that this is not contributing to their ongoing pathophysiology. This is particularly true in BMES.

CLINICS CARE POINTS

- Hypovitaminosis D is very common and does not correlate to age, sex, or socioeconomic status.
- All patients with significant fractures or arthrodesis should be placed on vitamin D and calcium supplementation (2000 IU/day + 1 gm/day, respectively).
- Patients with fragility fractures (low-energy injuries that would not be expected to cause a fracture) should be referred for workup for osteoporosis, because they are at increased risk for subsequent fractures.
- Although bone marrow edema syndrome, osteochondritis dissecans, and diabetic neuropathy have all been associated with increased hypovitaminosis D prevalence, no cause-and-effect relationship has been established.

DISCLOSURE

The author has nothing to disclose.

REFERENCES

1. Chevalley T, Brandi ML, Cashman KD, et al. Role of vitamin D supplementation in the management of musculoskeletal diseases: update from an European Society of Clinical and Economical Aspects of Osteoporosis, Osteoarthritis and Musculoskeletal Diseases (ESCEO) working group. Aging Clin Exp Res 2022;34(11):2603–23.
2. Sontag A, Krege JH. First fractures among postmenopausal women with osteoporosis. J Bone MinerMetab 2010;28(4):485–8.
3. Fischer V, Haffner-Luntzer M, Amling M, et al. Calcium and vitamin D in bone fracture healing and post-traumatic bone turnover. Eur Cell Mater 2018;35:365–85.
4. Holick MF. Vitamin D deficiency. N Engl J Med 2007;357(3):266–81.
5. Giakoumis M. The Impact of Vitamin D Levels in Foot and Ankle Surgery. Clin Podiatr Med Surg 2020;37(2):305–15.
6. Bernhard A, Matuk J. Vitamin D in Foot and Ankle Fracture Healing: A Literature Review and Research Design. Foot Ankle Spec 2015;8(5):397–405.
7. St Arnaud R, Naja RP. Vitamin D metabolism, cartilage and bone fracture repair. Mol Cell Endocrinol 2011;347(1–2):48–54.
8. Holick MF, Binkley NC, Bischoff-Ferrari HA, et al. Evaluation, treatment, and prevention of vitamin

D deficiency: an Endocrine Society clinical practice guideline. J Clin Endocrinol Metab 2011;96(7): 1911–30.

9. Gozdzik A, Barta JL, Wu H, et al. Low wintertime vitamin D levels in a sample of healthy young adults of diverse ancestry living in the Toronto area: associations with vitamin D intake and skin pigmentation. BMC Publ Health 2008;8:336.

10. Warner SJ, Garner MR, Nguyen JT, et al. Perioperative vitamin D levels correlate with clinical outcomes after ankle fracture fixation. Arch Orthop Trauma Surg 2016;136(3):339–44.

11. Smith JT, Halim K, Palms DA, et al. Prevalence of vitamin D deficiency in patients with foot and ankle injuries. Foot Ankle Int 2014;35(1):8–13.

12. Ribbans WJ, Aujla RS, Ashour R, et al. Vitamin D and foot and ankle trauma: An individual or societal problem. Foot 2019;39:100–5.

13. Bogunovic L, Kim AD, Beamer BS, et al. Hypovitaminosis D in patients scheduled to undergo orthopaedic surgery: a single-center analysis. JBone Joint SurgAm 2010;92(13):2300–4.

14. Michelson JD, Charlson MD. Vitamin D Status in an Elective Orthopedic Surgical Population. Foot Ankle Int 2016;37(2):186–91.

15. Kuriacose R, Olive KE. Prevalence of vitamin D deficiency and insufficiency in northeast Tennessee. South Med J 2008;101(9):906–9.

16. Stoker GE, Buchowski JM, Bridwell KH, et al. Preoperative vitamin D status of adults undergoing surgical spinal fusion. Spine (Phila Pa 1976) 2013; 38(6):507–15.

17. Bischoff-Ferrari HA, Can U, Staehelin HB, et al. Severe vitamin D deficiency in Swiss hip fracture patients. Bone 2008;42(3):597–602.

18. Sprague S, Petrisor B, Scott T, et al. What Is the Role of Vitamin D Supplementation in Acute Fracture Patients? A Systematic Review and Meta-Analysis of the Prevalence of Hypovitaminosis D and Supplementation Efficacy. J Orthop Trauma 2016;30(2):53–63.

19. Hanley DA, Davison KS. Vitamin D insufficiency in North America. JNutr 2005;135(2):332–7.

20. Chapuy MC, Preziosi P, Maamer M, et al. Prevalence of vitamin D insufficiency in an adult normal population. Osteoporos Int 1997;7(5):439–43.

21. Hagenau T, Vest R, Gissel TN, et al. Global vitamin D levels in relation to age, gender, skin pigmentation and latitude: an ecologic meta-regression analysis. Osteoporos Int 2009;20(1):133–40.

22. Fraissler L, Boelch SP, Schäfer T, et al. Vitamin D Deficiency in Patients With Idiopathic and Traumatic Osteochondritis Dissecans of the Talus. Foot Ankle Int 2019;40(11):1309–18.

23. Aujla RS, Allen PE, Ribbans WJ. Vitamin D levels in 577 consecutive elective foot & ankle surgery patients. Foot Ankle Surg 2019;25(3):310–5.

24. Plotnikoff GA, Quigley JM. Prevalence of severe hypovitaminosis D in patients with persistent, nonspecific musculoskeletal pain. Mayo Clin Proc 2003;78(12):1463–70.

25. Oberti V, Sanchez Ortiz M, Allende V, et al. Prevalence of hypovitaminosis D in patients with juvenile osteochondritis dissecans. Rev Esp Cir Ortop Traumatol (Engl Ed) 2021;65(2):132–7. Prevalencia de hipovitaminosis D en pacientes con osteocondritis disecante juvenil.

26. Mitchell DM, Henao MP, Finkelstein JS, et al. Prevalence and predictors of vitamin D deficiency in healthy adults. Endocr Pract 2012;18(6):914–23.

27. Barake R, Weiler H, Payette H, et al. Vitamin D status in healthy free-living elderly men and women living in Quebec, Canada. J Am Coll Nutr 2010; 29(1):25–30.

28. Bee CR, Sheerin DV, Wuest TK, et al. Serum vitamin D levels in orthopaedic trauma patients living in the northwestern United States. JOrthopTrauma 2013; 27(5):e103–6.

29. Williams BR, Thomas AJ, Collier RC, et al. Vitamin D Levels Do Not Predict Risk of Metatarsal Fractures. Foot Ankle Spec 2018;11(1):37–43.

30. Pellicane AJ, Wysocki NM, Schnitzer TJ. Prevalence of 25-hydroxyvitamin D deficiency in the outpatient rehabilitation population. Am J Phys Med Rehabil 2010;89(11):899–904.

31. Ginde AA, Liu MC, Camargo CA Jr. Demographic differences and trends of vitamin D insufficiency in the US population, 1988-2004. Arch Intern Med 2009;169(6):626–32.

32. Litwic A, Edwards M, Cooper C, et al. Geographic differences in fractures among women. Womens Health (Lond Engl) 2012;8(6):673–84.

33. Looker AC, Johnson CL, Lacher DA, et al. Vitamin D status: United States, 2001-2006. NCHSData Brief 2011;(59):1–8.

34. Amrein K, Scherkl M, Hoffmann M, et al. Vitamin D deficiency 2.0: an update on the current status worldwide. Eur J Clin Nutr 2020;74(11):1498–513.

35. Zalneraitis BH, Huuki E, Benavides LC, et al. Relation of Vitamin D Level, BMI, and Location of Lower Extremity Stress Fractures in Military Trainees. Mil Med 2022. https://doi.org/10.1093/milmed/usac258.

36. Seitz S, Koehne T, Ries C, et al. Impaired bone mineralization accompanied by low vitamin D and secondary hyperparathyroidism in patients with femoral neck fracture. Osteoporos Int 2013;24(2): 641–9.

37. Priemel M, von Domarus C, Klatte TO, et al. Bone mineralization defects and vitamin D deficiency: histomorphometric analysis of iliac crest bone biopsies and circulating 25-hydroxyvitamin D in 675 patients. J Bone Miner Res 2010;25(2):305–12.

38. Lewiecki EM, Bellido T, Bilezikian JP, et al. Proceedings of the 2023 Santa Fe bone symposium:

Progress and controversies in the management of patients with skeletal diseases. J Clin Densitom 2023;26(4):101432.

39. Cardoso DV, Veljkovic A. General Considerations About Foot and Ankle Arthrodesis. Any Way to Improve Our Results? Foot Ankle Clin 2022;27(4):701–22.

40. Childs BR, Andres BA, Vallier HA. Economic Benefit of Calcium and Vitamin D Supplementation: Does It Outweigh the Cost of Nonunions? J Orthop Trauma 2016;30(8):e285–8.

41. Andres BA, Childs BR, Vallier HA. Treatment of Hypovitaminosis D in an Orthopaedic Trauma Population. J Orthop Trauma 2018;32(4):e129–33.

42. Bodendorfer BMCJ, Robertson DS, Della Rocca GJ, et al. Do 25-Hydroxyvitamin D Levels Correlate With Fracture Complications? J Orthop Trauma 2016;30(9):e312–7.

43. Avenell A, Mak JC, O'Connell D. Vitamin D and vitamin D analogues for preventing fractures in post-menopausal women and older men. Cochrane Database Syst Rev 2014;2014(4):Cd000227.

44. Trivedi DP, Doll R, Khaw KT. Effect of four monthly oral vitamin D3 (cholecalciferol) supplementation on fractures and mortality in men and women living in the community: randomised double blind controlled trial. Bmj 2003;326(7387):469.

45. Myung SK, Cho H. Effects of intermittent or single high-dose vitamin D supplementation on risk of falls and fractures: a systematic review and meta-analysis. Osteoporos Int 2023;34(8):1355–67.

46. Marchand D, Loshak H. Duration of Bisphosphonate Treatment for Patients with Osteoporosis: A Review of Clinical Effectiveness and Guidelines. 2019. CADTH Rapid Response Reports.

47. Qutubuddin A, Cifu DX, Adler RA, et al. A pilot study of vitamin D and balance characteristics in middle-aged, healthy individuals. PMR 2010;2(1):23–6.

48. Krege JH, Wan X. Teriparatide and the risk of non-vertebral fractures in women with postmenopausal osteoporosis. Bone 2012;50(1):161–4.

49. Omeroglu S, Erdogan D, Omeroglu H. Effects of single high-dose vitamin D3 on fracture healing. An ultrastructural study in healthy guinea pigs. ArchOrthopTrauma Surg 1997;116(1–2):37–40.

50. Delgado-Martinez AD, Martinez ME, Carrascal MT, et al. Effect of 25-OH-vitamin D on fracture healing in elderly rats. J Orthop Res 1998;16(6):650–3.

51. Copp DH, Greenberg DM. Studies on Bone Fracture Healing I. Effect of Vitamins A and D. J Nutr 1945;4:261–7.

52. Omeroglu H, Ates Y, Akkus O, et al. Biomechanical analysis of the effects of single high-dose vitamin D3 on fracture healing in a healthy rabbit model. ArchOrthopTrauma Surg 1997;116(5):271–4.

53. Fu L, Tang T, Miao Y, et al. Effect of 1,25-dihydroxy vitamin D3 on fracture healing and bone remodeling in ovariectomized rat femora. Bone 2009;44(5):893–8.

54. Doetsch AM, Faber J, Lynnerup N, et al. The effect of calcium and vitamin D3 supplementation on the healing of the proximal humerus fracture: a randomized placebo-controlled study. Calcif Tissue Int 2004;75(3):183–8.

55. Ramanathan D, Emara AK, Pinney S, et al. Vitamin D Deficiency and Outcomes After Ankle Fusion: A Short Report. Foot Ankle Int 2022;43(5):703–5.

56. Moore KR, Howell MA, Saltrick KR, et al. Risk Factors Associated With Nonunion After Elective Foot and Ankle Reconstruction: A Case-Control Study. J Foot Ankle Surg 2017;56(3):457–62.

57. Brinker MR, O'Connor DP, Monla YT, et al. Metabolic and endocrine abnormalities in patients with nonunions. J Orthop Trauma 2007;21(8):557–70.

58. Chakhtoura M, Bacha DS, Gharios C, et al. Vitamin D Supplementation and Fractures in Adults: A Systematic Umbrella Review of Meta-Analyses of Controlled Trials. J Clin Endocrinol Metab 2022;107(3):882–98.

59. Russo K, Hallare D, Lee D, et al. Comparative Clinical Effects and Risk Factors Associated with Vitamin D in Foot and Ankle Fracture and Arthrodesis Healing. J Foot Ankle Surg 2023. https://doi.org/10.1053/j.jfas.2023.10.005.

60. Boszczyk AM, Zakrzewski P, Pomianowski S. Vitamin D concentration in patients with normal and impaired bone union. PolOrthopTraumatol 2013;78(1–3):1–3.

61. Gorter EA, Hamdy NA, Appelman-Dijkstra NM, et al. The role of vitamin D in human fracture healing: a systematic review of the literature. Bone 2014;64:288–97.

62. Lappe J, Cullen D, Haynatzki G, et al. Calcium and vitamin d supplementation decreases incidence of stress fractures in female navy recruits. J Bone Miner Res 2008;23(5):741–9.

63. Richards T, Wright C. British Army recruits with low serum vitamin D take longer to recover from stress fractures. BMJ Mil Health 2020;166(4):240–2.

64. Miller JR, Dunn KW, Ciliberti LJ Jr, et al. Association of Vitamin D With Stress Fractures: A Retrospective Cohort Study. J Foot Ankle Surg 2016;55(1):117–20.

65. McCabe MP, Smyth MP, Richardson DR. Current concept review: vitamin D and stress fractures. Foot Ankle Int 2012;33(6):526–33.

66. Pereira Filho MV, Stéfani KC, Ferreira GF, et al. Risk Factors Associated With Foot and Ankle Insufficiency Fractures in Postmenopausal Sedentary Women. Foot Ankle Int 2021;42(4):482–7.

67. Cohn MR, Gianakos AL, Grueter K, et al. Update on the Comprehensive Approach to Fragility Fractures. J Orthop Trauma 2018;32(9):480–90.

68. 2023. Available at: https://frax-tool.org/. Accessed November 29, 2023.

69. Greenhagen RM, Frykberg RG, Wukich DK. Serum vitamin D and diabetic foot complications. Diabet Foot Ankle 2019;10(1):1579631.

70. Greenhagen RM, Wukich DK, Jung RH, et al. Peripheral and central bone mineral density in Charcot's neuroarthropathy compared in diabetic and nondiabetic populations. J Am Podiatr Med Assoc 2012;102(3):213–22.

71. Petrova NL, Donaldson NK, Bates M, et al. Effect of Recombinant Human Parathyroid Hormone (1-84) on Resolution of Active Charcot Neuroosteoarthropathy in Diabetes: A Randomized, Double-Blind, Placebo-Controlled Study. Diabetes Care 2021;44(7):1613–21.

72. Maier GS, Lazovic D, Maus U, et al. Vitamin D Deficiency: The Missing Etiological Factor in the Development of Juvenile Osteochondrosis Dissecans? J Pediatr Orthop 2019;39(1):51–4.

73. Eidmann A, Eisert M, Rudert M, et al. Influence of Vitamin D and C on Bone Marrow Edema Syndrome-A Scoping Review of the Literature. J Clin Med 2022;11(22). https://doi.org/10.3390/jcm11226820.

74. Oehler N, Mussawy H, Schmidt T, et al. Identification of vitamin D and other bone metabolism parameters as risk factors for primary bone marrow oedema syndrome. BMC Musculoskelet Disord 2018;19(1):451.

75. Horas K, Fraissler L, Maier G, et al. High Prevalence of Vitamin D Deficiency in Patients With Bone Marrow Edema Syndrome of the Foot and Ankle. Foot Ankle Int 2017;38(7):760–6.

76. Sprinchorn AE, O'Sullivan R, Beischer AD. Transient bone marrow edema of the foot and ankle and its association with reduced systemic bone mineral density. Foot Ankle Int 2011;32(5):S508–12.

Surgical Outcomes in Charcot Arthropathy

William C. Skinner, MD[a], Naveen Pattisapu, MD[b], Jane Yeoh, MD[c],
Benjamin J. Grear, MD[a], David R. Richardson, MD[a], Garnett A. Murphy, MD[a],
Clayton C. Bettin, MD[a,*]

KEYWORDS

- Charcot neuroarthropathy • Charcot arthropathy • Operative treatment • Foot and ankle
- Joint disease

KEY POINTS

- Charcot neuroarthropathy (CN) of the foot and ankle is a progressive disease process with destructive bony changes and oftentimes deformity which is most commonly seen in the setting of diabetes mellitus with peripheral neuropathy.
- Impaired bone healing and metabolism with decreased bone mineral density are of significant concern when managing patients with CN, particularly when surgical intervention is indicated.
- Operative treatment options include surgical debridement of ulcers, ostectomy, temporizing fixation, and deformity correction with arthrodesis.
- The goal of treatment is to maintain a plantigrade, ulcer-free foot.
- Surgical interventions may be indicated in the setting of infection, nonhealing ulceration with or without bony prominences, and/or progressive or unstable deformities.

INTRODUCTION

Charcot neuroarthropathy (CN) of the foot and ankle is well known in the orthopedic literature for its significant morbidity. The natural history of CN is one of progressive bone and joint destruction leading to potentially catastrophic alterations of the bony architecture of the foot and ankle with high rates of ulceration, infection, and ultimately limb amputation.

Originally, CN was described in the 1800s by Jean-Martin Charcot[1] who noted this destructive joint disease in patients with tertiary neurosyphilis. In modern times, the primary cause of CN of the foot is diabetes mellitus with peripheral neuropathy.[2] Most studies of diabetic populations support an incidence of less than 1% of developing CN, but several studies focusing on populations of diabetic patients with peripheral neuropathy have suggested the incidence may

be even higher.[3–5] Recent epidemiologic data published in 2019 estimated that 463 million individuals worldwide have been diagnosed with diabetes mellitus, and this is projected to increase to 578 million by 2030.[6]

In 2011, an international task force of experts produced a consensus report summarizing much of the current understanding of the Charcot foot. A diabetic patient with peripheral neuropathy is a susceptible individual for developing a Charcot process. Not all diabetic patients develop CN, but having diabetes with peripheral neuropathy is a predisposing factor. In these susceptible individuals, loss of protective peripheral sensation can lead to bone injury of the foot or ankle, and bone injury via either macrotrauma or microtrauma may trigger an increased or unregulated inflammatory cascade. The local proinflammatory state at the site of injury upregulates osteoclast function and favors osteolysis

---

[a] Campbell Clinic Department of Orthopaedic Surgery and Biomedical Engineering, University of Tennessee Health Science Center, 1211 Union Avenue, Suite 510, Memphis, TN 38104, USA; [b] Beth Israel Lahey Hospital, 41 Mall Road, Burlington, MA 01805, USA; [c] Nanaimo Orthopaedics, 201-1515 Dufferin Crescent, Nanaimo, British Columbia V9S5H6, Canada
* Corresponding author. Campbell Clinic Foundation, 1211 Union Avenue, Suite 510, Memphis, TN 38104.
E-mail address: cbettin@campbellclinic.com

Orthop Clin N Am 55 (2024) 393–401
https://doi.org/10.1016/j.ocl.2023.11.001
0030-5898/24/© 2023 Elsevier Inc. All rights reserved.

which can precipitate varying degrees of bone fragmentation and/or destruction. Additionally, autonomic dysfunction with vasodilation and hyperemia has been proposed as another mechanism potentially contributing to bone resorption.[7,8]

In general, treatment strategies for CN center around achieving a stable, plantigrade, ulcer-free foot.[9] Management may consist of nonoperative treatment with total contact casting (TCC), weight-bearing restrictions, and eventual transition to accommodative footwear.[10] TCC transfers and disperses 30% of the pressure to the cast wall, thus offloading the pressure points of the foot.[11] Even with the load sharing of a TCC, there still is a recurrence rate of 30% with regard to ulceration.[12] An alternative to TCC is the use of a Charcot restraint orthotic walker (CROW boot) that may allow for easier monitoring of ulcers if present.[13] Not all CNs respond to conservative measures, and operative treatment of CN may be indicated for chronic, recurrent, or impending ulcerations or in the face of a deformity that cannot be braced. Surgical interventions range from simple debridement to complex reconstructions and arthrodesis. Ulceration may be managed in a more limited fashion with surgical debridement, with or without exostectomy, followed by TCC.[14,15] With more advanced disease, though, deformity correction and arthrodesis often are needed.[16,17]

Charcot arthropathy of the foot and ankle negatively impacts patient quality of life.[8,18,19] A Finnish cohort of patients with CN of the foot or ankle, which included a mix of operatively and nonoperatively managed patients, showed significant reduction in quality of life outcome scores (36-Item Short Form Survey) compared with the general population controls. Furthermore, this cohort of patients with CN secondary to diabetes mellitus showed lower levels of SF-36 quality of life scores (physical functioning, role physical, social functioning, and general health) than chronically ill population controls as well.[18] Similarly, other studies have demonstrated that diabetics with CN have lower quality of life physical functioning scores than diabetics without CN.[19] Maintaining a stable, plantigrade foot that is free of ulceration may significantly impact quality of life outcomes in this population.

Few studies on medium to long-term outcomes after operative management of CN exist. Rates of postintervention ulceration, infection, and amputation are fundamental to guiding treatment strategies, but they are inconsistently reported in the literature. The purpose of this review is to summarize general outcomes related to the operative management of CN. Additionally, this article reviews long-term follow-up data (average 46 months) on 2 cohorts of patients with CN who have undergone operative intervention at a single tertiary referral institution. Surgical outcome data can be used to assist surgeons in counseling patients on expected outcomes and to serve as comparison for future studies of new surgical strategies.

PATIENT EVALUATION OVERVIEW

Diabetic foot complications (eg, infection, ulceration, Charcot arthropathy) carry significant morbidity and mortality, and the number of patients afflicted by this only continues to rise. It is estimated that 148 million diabetic patients will develop an ulcer in their lifetime, and 75 million will develop a diabetic foot infection.[20] In addition to glycemic management, a combination of routine foot care, evaluation, and counseling are essential preventative steps in combating this growing problem.[21]

When complications do arise, referral to an orthopedic foot and ankle specialist is paramount. A thorough history should elicit information such as glycemic control, functional status, review of shoe wear, history of ulceration, history of infection, previous treatments with nonoperative modalities, previous surgical intervention and/or wound care, and review of other comorbidities. A comprehensive foot and ankle examination should be performed at each visit. Of particular importance, the examiner should note the degree/location of sensory loss, skin changes, callosities, wounds/ulcers, presence/absence of infection, equinus contractures, deformities, and vascular status.[8,22]

Radiographic evaluation of the foot and ankle is an essential part of the new patient workup but should also be obtained when an established patient develops a new problem or examination finding (eg, pain, erythema, edema, deformity). Radiographs may reveal normal bony anatomy or demonstrate significant destruction of the foot and/or ankle joints consistent with CN. Poor bone quality is also frequently encountered in the setting of diabetic foot disease and should also be documented, as this will factor into treatment decisions.[23]

Additional laboratory workup may be indicated depending on the patient's diagnosis and previous information provided at the time of referral. Obtaining a recent hemoglobin A1c applies to the management of all diabetic patients. In patients with fracture or concern for bone healing/health such as diabetic patients, it is reasonable to obtain a vitamin D level and provide supplementation as appropriate.[24] For infection, the provider should consider obtaining a complete blood count, erythrocyte sedimentation rate, and C-reactive protein both to aid in diagnosis and monitor treatment response.[25,26]

Charcot arthropathy may be suspected on initial evaluation, but the diagnosis can be confirmed with radiographs. These may range from minor bone fragmentation with maintained joint alignment to severe collapse or erosion with total loss of joint space and alignment.[27,28] Occasionally, radiographs may appear benign, but a diabetic patient with significant edema, erythema, and low concern for infection may be experiencing an early Charcot process.[29,30]

Once diagnosed with CN, treatment options depend on many factors. The surgeon must consider the type of deformity, location of deformity, chronicity, presence of ulcers, presence of infection, glycemic control, tissue perfusion/vascular status, bone quality, functional status, and smoking status when weighing recommendations for nonoperative versus operative management.

NONPHARMACOLOGIC OR SURGICAL/INTERVENTIONAL TREATMENT OPTIONS

The Eichenholtz classification divides the progression of CN into 3 stages and is still widely used today. Eichenholtz stage 1, otherwise known as the fragmentation phase, represents the acute injury stage where radiographs may demonstrate osteopenia, joint subluxation, and/or bony fragmentation/fracture. As the disease process continues, the acute inflammatory phase transitions to a process of early repair. This is referred to as Eichenholtz stage 2 or the coalescence phase. On clinical examination, less swelling, erythema, and warmth is noted and radiographic changes such as healing of fragmented bone, resorption of bony debris, and sclerosis may be seen which are consistent with stage 2 disease. In Eichenholtz stage 3, inflammation has subsided, and evidence of remodeling predominates though significant deformity may be present depending on the degree of bone destruction and subsequent loss of alignment that occurred in earlier stages. Radiographs during this stage demonstrate arthrosis of the involved areas with subchondral sclerosis, osteophytic changes, and loss of joint space. Eichenholtz stage 0 has been added to the classification to describe the earliest phase of the disease where only clinical examination suggests

a Charcot process (swelling, erythema, warmth, and other symptoms) and infection has been ruled out, but radiographs are still normal.[31,32]

When discussing Eichenholtz stage I disease, immobilization and weight-bearing limitations have been mainstays of treatment once an acute Charcot process is diagnosed. The goal is to minimize destructive changes and maintain a plantigrade foot while the acute, inflammatory process runs its course. Recent data suggest that TCC with weight-bearing permitted in the cast and frequent cast changes are reasonable treatment strategies for patients with stage I disease without significant deformity.[33–35] CROW is another described form of immobilization for management that has been utilized with good results.[13,36]

Though many patients can avoid surgery and return to accommodative shoe wear with or without orthoses, this strategy of treatment may come at a cost. A study of patients with CN treated with TCC and offloading showed significant decreases in bone mineral density after treatment compared with patients with neuropathic ulcers without CN treated with the same modalities. At the conclusion of the treatment, 84% of the CN feet included were classified as osteopenic or osteoporotic.[37]

The most limited surgical intervention (LSI) is debridement of nonhealing ulcers or infected soft tissue. Soft tissue debridements may be performed in isolation or may be combined with partial resection of bone depending on the pathologic anatomy or presence of underlying osteomyelitis. Commonly, debridement and exostectomy are performed for chronic ulceration of the Charcot foot that has failed extensive conservative treatment. Studies have demonstrated successful short-term results with regard to ulcer resolution and wound healing in patients managed with exostectomy. Despite high rates of ulcer resolution typically within 6 to 10 weeks after debridement and resection of bony exostoses, patients remain at high risk for recurrence of ulceration or developing new areas of ulceration with longer term follow-up.[10,15,38]

In patients with more significant or progressive deformities, major reconstructive type procedures are often indicated. The goal of reconstructive procedures is to achieve a stable, plantigrade foot and decrease the lifetime risk of ulceration and infection which can lead to amputation. This is accomplished through osteotomies and/or bone resection to correct the rigid deformity and arthrodesis to maintain correction. Due to the heterogeneity of patient factors and location of the deformity, there are many variations of reconstructive procedures described in the literature for the Charcot foot or ankle.

Deformity correction can be stabilized internally, externally, or using a hybrid of these fixation types. External fixation typically refers to application of a ring/circular static frame, which is applied in a manner to maintain the corrected deformity and achieve bony fusion. Proponents of external fixation for arthrodesis in the treatment of CN deformities point to smaller surgical wounds, less reliance on bone quality for fixation, and ability to perform single-stage reconstruction in the presence of infection as theoretic advantages.[22] In a large retrospective series, Pinzur and colleagues[39] achieved a plantigrade, noninfected foot in approximately 95% of CN patients who underwent single-stage resection of osteomyelitis, deformity correction, and application of a static ringed external fixator. Rates of minor and major complications with external fixation are high. These range from cellulitis and pin-site infections, which are most common, to more significant complications such as peri-implant fracture, nonunion, deep infection, and/or loss of correction.[40]

Internal fixation using plates, screws, and intramedullary devices for CN reconstruction of the foot and ankle has been widely described (Fig. 1A–C). Theoretic advantages of internal fixation include lower rates of superficial infections, less patient burden compared with a frame (pin-site care, frame prominence, social stigma, and so forth), and improved fixation techniques. Overall, there is limited evidence directly comparing internal fixation and external fixation, and major endpoints of postoperative outcomes between these techniques are similar in the current literature. When considering reconstructive procedures overall, there is a wide range of reported outcomes. A current review of CN surgical outcomes reveals postoperative infection rates ranging from 0% to 50% and rates of recurrent ulceration from 0% to 25%.[41–47] Reported amputation rates similarly vary widely from 0% to 42.8%.[48–51] In a 2016 systematic review, Schneekloth and colleagues[52] included 30 studies (860 patients) pertaining to the operative management of CN. The heterogeneity of included studies limited the assessment of outcomes, but they reported a cumulative major amputation rate of 8.9% (77 of 860) among studies reviewed.[52]

Previously unpublished data on the operative management of CN at our institution showed similar outcomes to the ranges of postoperative infection, recurrent ulceration, and amputation that have been reported. Fifty-eight patients with CN who were treated surgically over a period of 11 years (November 2005 to May 2017), with an average follow-up of 46 months, were retrospectively reviewed. The patients were divided into 2 groups for analysis based on the type of surgical intervention: 32 patients

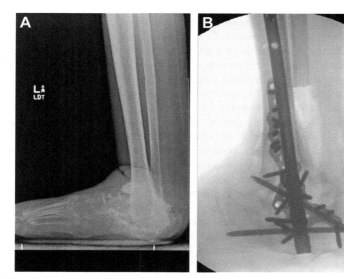
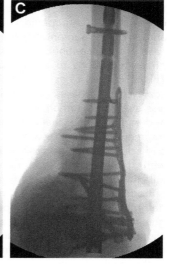

Fig. 1. Example of Charcot neuroarthropathy (CN) reconstruction with internal fixation. (A) Preoperative lateral radiograph of a patient with Charcot neuropathy of the ankle and hindfoot with significant deformity. (B) Lateral fluoroscopic image after tibiotalocalcaneal arthrodesis with an intramedullary nail and locking plate construct for the treatment of CN. (C) Anteroposterior ankle fluoroscopic image after tibiotalocalcaneal arthrodesis with an intramedullary nail and locking plate construct for treatment of CN.

underwent LSI, and 26 patients underwent reconstructive surgery (RS). LSI entailed debridement and irrigation, exostectomy, temporizing external fixation, open reduction internal fixation not associated with arthrodesis, or minor or major amputation (without prior operative management of CN). RS included arthrodesis procedures with different types of fixation methods (intramedullary nails, plates, and external fixators) as chosen by the operative surgeon. This series did not include superconstructs in the RS cohort. Postintervention infection and recurrent ulceration occurred in a substantial percentage of patients after LSI and RS (25% and 42% infection and 34% and 42% ulceration, respectively). Over 20% of patients went on to have an amputation regardless of the type of surgery (LSI group = 21.8%, RS group = 23.1%).

TREATMENT COMPLICATIONS

The operative management of CN is certainly noted to have significant rates of minor and major complications, but this can be misconstrued if discussed in isolation. CN typically occurs in diabetics who may have poor glycemic control and often 1 or more associated medical comorbidities such that population of study is already at an increased baseline risk for any surgical intervention. Poor bone quality is also of significant concern in the diabetic CN patient population and factors into discussion of fixation strategies as well as potential complications. When discussing the risks of intervention for an unstable Charcot process with the patient, it is imperative to also consider the natural history of the disease process and effectively communicate this to the patient. Developing an ulcer puts the patient at significantly increased risk of requiring amputation during their lifetime.

Minor Complications

- Superficial infection/pin-site infection
- Wound dehiscence
- Recurrent ulceration
- Hardware loosening without catastrophic failure

Major Complications

- Intraoperative/postoperative fracture
- Deep infection
- Loss of deformity correction
- Hardware failure
- Nonunion

One study reported the lifetime amputation rate after ulceration to be 20%, though other lower quality studies suggest this rate may be greater than 50%.[53,54] The operative management of CN does come with high complication rates, but the ultimate goal is to maintain or recreate a stable, plantigrade foot free of ulceration and lessen the lifetime risk of amputation.

EVALUATION OF OUTCOMES

Many outcomes are reported in the study of CN, though the most impactful of these are likely postintervention rates of recurrent ulceration, infection, and amputation. Additional outcomes such as patient-reported outcomes, quality of life scores, union rates, and others are important to consider, but, given the historically high rates of limb amputation, the focus of CN surgical intervention are the core metrics contributing to successful limb salvage (ie, minimizing wound recurrence and infection). Most studies on the operative management of CN reported on ulceration, infection, and amputation rates, but there is some variability in how these were reported which limits comparison. Infection in certain studies may have been classified as deep or superficial when reported in the analysis while others superficial infections may have been excluded entirely, and still in others deep and superficial infections were considered together in a single category of infection. The majority of studies clearly reported postintervention ulceration rates. Some studies reported these ulceration rates referring only to recurrence of the ulcer in the same location while others pooled recurrence of an ulcer and new ulcers in different locations of the foot or ankle into the same rate. Amputation rates are often reported as major or minor, but at times this may be presented in aggregate. This is important for evaluating outcomes because minor amputation such as toe amputation carries significantly less morbidity and functional limitation than major amputation such as transtibial amputation. Both are important to note, but differentiating between the 2 allows for more accurate assessment of outcomes.

NEW DEVELOPMENTS

Superconstructs are of continued interest in Charcot reconstruction procedures. Correction of large deformities in patients with poor bone quality warrants careful consideration of implant selection to maintain correction and ideally achieve union of the arthrodesis. As previously discussed, the pathophysiology of CN involves both sensory impairment and autonomic dysfunction. The bony

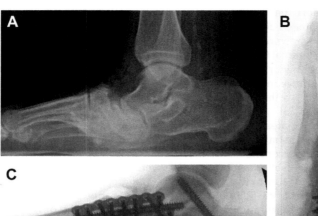
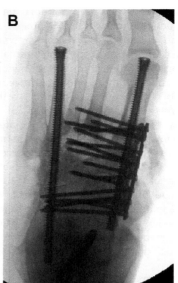
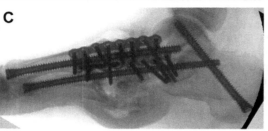

Fig. 2. Example of a midfoot superconstruct. (A) Preoperative lateral foot radiograph demonstrating midfoot Charcot neuroarthropathy (CN) with significant destructive changes and collapse. (B) Lateral fluoroscopic view of the foot after reconstruction with intramedullary beams and medial column locking plate. (C) Anteroposterior fluoroscopic view of the foot after reconstruction with intramedullary beams and medial column locking plate.

changes (dissolution, fragmentation, osteopenia, and so forth.) seen in the later stages of CN result from the combination of continued microtrauma, hyperemia, and dysregulated inflammatory cascade.[7,8] The abnormal bone encountered in CN reconstructive procedures poses fixation challenges.

Superconstructs are described in the literature with the following criteria: fusion extends beyond the zone of deformity to include uninvolved joints as a means of improving fixation, aggressive bone resection allows for deformity reduction without excess soft-tissue tension, use of the strongest device tolerated by the soft tissues, and maximizing the mechanical advantage of the implants to achieve stability.[52,55] Hybrid internal fixation constructs using intramedullary bolts or beams extending beyond the zone of deformity with supplementary locking plate fixation is an example of a superconstruct employed in the treatment of midfoot CN. In a study including 20 patients with midfoot CN with deformity, 95% of the patients reported a satisfactory result with a mean 2-year follow-up when treated with a midfoot superconstruct for reconstruction, and only 1 patient required amputation during the follow-up period.[56] Fixation strategies and implants continue to evolve and play an important role in improving outcomes in surgical reconstruction for CN.

At the authors' institution, midfoot superconstructs (intramedullary bolts or beams with medial column locking plates) have been used for the treatment of CN since January 2017 and have shown potential benefit (Fig. 2A–C). Compared with baseline institutional controls on reconstructive procedures for CN (not including superconstructs), these midfoot superconstructs have shown a 25% reduction in postoperative ulceration rate, 43% reduction in postoperative deep infection rate, and 31% reduction in major amputation.

SUMMARY/FUTURE DIRECTIONS

CN is a progressive disease process with high rates of complications and treatment failures. Operative intervention for CN ranges from limited debridements to complex reconstructions which aim to alter the natural history of this disease process by minimizing traditionally high rates of ulceration, deep infection, and amputation. Large prospective studies of the operative management of CN are difficult to conduct, and the majority of evidence comes from retrospective case series. Furthermore, there is a significant amount of heterogeneity in patient factors, interventions, and studied outcomes which at times limits comparisons of existing treatments.

To improve patient outcomes, areas of future study may further examine.

- Modifications to traditional constructs and/ or application of existing fixation devices

- Direct comparisons of internal and external fixation strategies for reconstructive procedures in CN
- Superconstructs for reconstructive procedures in CN
- Prevention/diabetic education and management
- Early versus delayed reconstruction
- Application of biologics/wound-healing strategies
- Bone metabolism, bone repair, and improving bone health in diabetic patients

CLINIC CARE POINTS

- The prevalence of diabetic CN of the foot and ankle has been reported from 0.08% to 13.0%, though most studies suggest it is in the lower end of this range.[4]
- Decreased bone mineral density is of significant concern when treating CN with 84% of feet categorized as osteopenic or osteoporotic after conservative management with TCC.[37]
- Treatment of CN aims to maintain a plantigrade foot free of ulceration, and surgical intervention often plays a role in treatment when conservative measures fail or significant deformity is present.[8]
- Reported major amputation rates after RS for CN range significantly from 0% up to 42.8% in small case series, though a systematic review found a cumulative major amputation rate of 8.9%.[51,52]
- Hybrid internal fixation constructs and superconstructs are becoming more common when performing reconstructive procedures for CN where bone quality is often poor. This is an area of continued study with good results at midterm follow-up.[56]

DISCLOSURE

The authors have no relevant disclosures.

REFERENCES

1. Charcot JM. Lecons sur, les maladies du système nerveux. New York, USA: Cambridge University Press; 1886.
2. Zgonis T, Roukis TS, Lamm BM. Charcot foot and ankle reconstruction: current thinking and surgical approaches. Clin Podiatr Med Surg 2007;24(3):505–17.
3. Sinha S, Munichoodappa CS, Kozak GP. Neuroarthropathy (Charcot joints) in diabetes mellitus (clinical study of 101 cases). Medicine 1972;51(3):191–210.
4. Frykberg RG, Belczyk R. Epidemiology of the Charcot foot. Clin Podiatr Med Surg 2008;25(1):17–28.
5. Cofield RH, Morrison MJ, Beabout JW. Diabetic neuroarthropathy in the foot: patient characteristics and patterns of radiographic change. Foot Ankle 1983;4(1):15–22.
6. Saeedi P, Petersohn I, Salpea P, et al. Global and regional diabetes prevalence estimates for 2019 and projections for 2030 and 2045: Results from the International Diabetes Federation Diabetes Atlas. Diabetes Res Clin Pract 2019;157:107843.
7. Rogers LC, Frykberg RG, Armstrong DG, et al. The Charcot foot in diabetes. J Am Podiatr Med Assoc 2011;101(5):437–46.
8. Strotman PK, Reif TJ, Pinzur MS. Charcot arthropathy of the foot and ankle. Foot Ankle Int 2016;37(11):1255–63.
9. Johnson JE. Operative treatment of neuropathic arthropathy of the foot and ankle. J Bone Joint Surg Am 1998;80(11):1700.
10. Wukich DK, Sung W. Charcot arthropathy of the foot and ankle: modern concepts and management review. J Diabetes Complications 2009;23(6):409–26.
11. Shaw JE, Hsi W-L, Ulbrecht JS, et al. The mechanism of plantar unloading in total contact casts: implications for design and clinical use. Foot Ankle Int 1997;18(12):809–17.
12. Guyton GP. An analysis of iatrogenic complications from the total contact cast. Foot Ankle Int 2005;26(11):903–7.
13. Mehta JA, Brown C, Sargeant N. Charcot restraint orthotic walker. Foot Ankle Int 1998;19(9):619–23.
14. Catanzariti AR, Mendicino R, Haverstock B. Ostectomy for diabetic neuroarthropathy involving the midfoot. J Foot Ankle Surg 2000;39(5):291–300.
15. Laurinaviciene R, Kirketerp-Moller K, Holstein P. Exostectomy for chronic midfoot plantar ulcer in Charcot deformity. J Wound Care 2008;17(2):53–8.
16. Mueller MJ, Sinacore DR, Hastings MK, et al. Effect ofAchilles tendon lengthening on neuropathic plantar ulcers*: a randomized clinical trial. J Bone Joint Surg Am 2003;85(8):1436–45.
17. Pinzur MS. Current concepts review: Charcot arthropathy of the foot and ankle. Foot Ankle Int 2007;28(8):952–9.
18. Pakarinen T-K, Laine H-J, Mäenpää H, et al. Long-term outcome and quality of life in patients with Charcot foot. Foot Ankle Surg 2009;15(4):187–91.
19. Dhawan V, Spratt KF, Pinzur MS, et al. Reliability of AOFAS diabetic foot questionnaire in Charcot arthropathy: stability, internal consistency, and measurable difference. Foot Ankle Int 2005;26(9):717–31.

20. Chastain CA, Klopfenstein N, Serezani CH, et al. A clinical review of diabetic foot infections. Clin Podiatr Med Surg 2019;36(3):381–95.

21. Ortegon MM, Redekop WK, Niessen LW. Cost-effectiveness of prevention and treatment of the diabetic foot: a Markov analysis. Diabetes Care 2004;27(4):901–7.

22. Pinzur MS. The diabetic foot and neuroarthropathy. In: Coughlin MJ, Mann RA, Saltzman CL, editors. Surgery of the foot and ankle. 10th edition. Philadelphia, PA: Elsevier; 2023. p. 1330–71.

23. Rabe OC, Winther-Jensen M, Allin KH, et al. Fractures and osteoporosis in patients with diabetes with Charcot foot. Diabetes Care 2021;44(9):2033–8.

24. Yoho RM, Frerichs J, Dodson NB, et al. A comparison of vitamin D levels in nondiabetic and diabetic patient populations. JJ Am Podiatr Med Assoc 2009;99(1):35–41.

25. Lavery LA, Ahn J, Ryan EC, et al. What are the optimal cutoff values for ESR and CRP to diagnose osteomyelitis in patients with diabetes-related foot infections? Clin Orthop Relat Res 2019;477(7):1594.

26. Armstrong DG, Tan T-W, Boulton AJ, et al. Diabetic Foot Ulcers: A Review. JAMA 2023;330(1):62–75.

27. Eichenholtz S. Charcot joints. Springfield (IL): Charles C Thomas; 1966.

28. Rosenbaum AJ, DiPreta JA. Classifications in brief: Eichenholtz classification of Charcot arthropathy. Clin Orthop Relat Res 2015;473(3):1168–71.

29. Shibata T, Tada K, Hashizume C. The results of arthrodesis of the ankle for leprotic neuroarthropathy. J Bone Joint Surg Am 1990;72(5):749–56.

30. Sella EJ, Barrette C. Staging of Charcot neuroarthropathy along the medial column of the foot in the diabetic patient. J Foot Ankle Surg 1999;38(1):34–40.

31. van der Ven A, Chapman CB, Bowker JH. Charcot neuropathy of the Foot and Ankle. J Am Acad Orthop Surg 2009;17:562–71.

32. Dodd A, Daniels TR. Charcot neuropathy of the foot and ankle. J Bone Joint Surg Am 2018;100:696–711.

33. Pinzur MS, Lio T, Posner M. Treatment of Eichenholtz stage I Charcot foot arthropathy with a weightbearing total contact cast. Foot Ankle Int 2006;27(5):324–9.

34. Pinzur M. Surgical versus accommodative treatment for Charcot arthropathy of the midfoot. Foot Ankle Int 2004;25(8):545–9.

35. de Souza LJ. Charcot arthropathy and immobilization in a weight-bearing total contact cast. J Bone Joint Surg Am 2008;90(4):754–9.

36. Morgan JM, Biehl WC 3rd, Wagner FW Jr. Management of neuropathic arthropathy with the Charcot Restraint Orthotic Walker. Clin Orthop Relat Res 1993;296:58–63.

37. Sinacore DR, Hastings MK, Bohnert KL, et al. Immobilization-induced osteolysis and recovery in neuropathic foot impairments. Bone 2017;105:237–44.

38. Brodsky JW, Rouse AM. Exostectomy for symptomatic bony prominences in diabetic Charcot feet. Clin Orthop Rel Res 1993;296:21–6.

39. Pinzur MS, Gil J, Belmares J. Treatment of osteomyelitis in charcot foot with single-stage resection of infection, correction of deformity, and maintenance with ring fixation. Foot Ankle Int 2012;33(12):1069–74.

40. Lowery NJ, Woods JB, Armstrong DG, et al. Surgical management of Charcot neuroarthropathy of the foot and ankle: a systematic review. Foot Ankle Int 2012;33(2):113–21.

41. Cullen BD, Weinraub GM, Van Gompel G. Early results with use of the midfoot fusion bolt in Charcot arthropathy. J Foot Ankle Surg 2013;52(2):235–8.

42. Ford SE, Cohen BE, Davis WH, et al. Clinical outcomes and complications of midfoot Charcot reconstruction with intramedullary beaming. Foot Ankle Int 2019;40(1):18–23.

43. Garchar D, DiDomenico LA, Klaue K. Reconstruction of Lisfranc joint dislocations secondary to Charcot neuroarthropathy using a plantar plate. J Foot Ankle Surg 2013;52(3):295–7.

44. Grant WP, Garcia-Lavin S, Sabo R. Beaming the columns for Charcot diabetic foot reconstruction: a retrospective analysis. J Foot Ankle Surg 2011;50(2):182–9.

45. Richter M, Mittlmeier T, Rammelt S, et al. Intramedullary fixation in severe Charcot osteoneuroarthropathy with foot deformity results in adequate correction without loss of correction– Results from a multi-centre study. Foot Ankle Surg 2015;21(4):269–76.

46. Mehlhorn AT, Walther M, Iblher N, et al. Complication assessment and prevention strategies using midfoot fusion bolt for medial column stabilization in Charcot's osteoarthropathy. Foot 2016;29:36–41.

47. Wiewiorski M, Yasui T, Miska M, et al. Solid bolt fixation of the medial column in Charcot midfoot arthropathy. J Foot Ankle Surg 2013;52(1):88–94.

48. DeVries JG, Berlet GC, Hyer CF. A retrospective comparative analysis of Charcot ankle stabilization using an intramedullary rod with or without application of circular external fixator—utilization of the Retrograde Arthrodesis Intramedullary Nail database. J Foot Ankle Surg 2012;51(4):420–5.

49. Dos Santos-Vaquinhas A, Parra G, Martínez P, et al. Beaming in the Charcot foot: A case series with 12-month minimum follow-up. Foot 2021;47:101814.

50. Eschler A, Wussow A, Ulmar B, et al. Intramedullary medial column support with the Midfoot Fusion Bolt (MFB) is not sufficient for osseous healing of arthrodesis in neuroosteoarthropathic feet. Injury 2014;45:S38–43.

51. Safavi PS, Jupiter DC, Panchbhavi V. A systematic review of current surgical interventions for Charcot

neuroarthropathy of the midfoot. J Foot Ankle Surg 2017;56(6):1249–52.

52. Schneekloth BJ, Lowery NJ, Wukich DK. Charcot neuroarthropathy in patients with diabetes: an updated systematic review of surgical management. J Foot Ankle Surg 2016;55(3):586–90.

53. Edmonds M, Manu C, Vas P. The current burden of diabetic foot disease. J Clin Orthop Trauma 2021; 17:88–93.

54. Narres M, Kvitkina T, Claessen H, et al. Incidence of lower extremity amputations in the diabetic compared with the non-diabetic population: a systematic review. PLoS One 2017;12(8):e0182081.

55. Sammarco VJ. Superconstructs in the treatment of Charcot foot deformity: plantar plating, locked plating, and axial screw fixation. Foot Ankle Clin 2009;14(3):393–407.

56. Frøkjær J. Surgical treatment of midfoot charcot neuroarthropathy review of literature and our results after superconstruct reconstruction of midfoot charcot neuroarthropathy. J Clin Orthop Trauma 2021;17:59–64.

Spine

Treatment Strategies in the Osteoporotic Spine

Daniel Gelvez, MD[a],*, Katherine Dong, MD[a], Nathan Redlich, MD[a],
Jestin Williams, MD[a], Amit Bhandutia, MD[a], Berje Shamassian, MD[b]

KEYWORDS

• Spine surgery • Osteoporosis • Instrumentation • Vertebral compression fractures

---

KEY POINTS

- Osteoporosis directly leads to spinal pathology, including deformity and vertebral compression fractures. It requires careful patient selection, evaluation, optimization, and surgical planning.
- Patients evaluated by spine surgeons should be screened for osteoporosis with appropriate laboratory work and imaging, and should be optimized for surgery with appropriate medical treatment to maximize bone quality.
- Surgical techniques including increased points of fixation, modification of instrumentation techniques, and cement augmentation can be employed to obtain successful surgical outcomes.
- Vertebral compression fractures can be managed operatively and nonoperatively. Treatment plan should be patient specific.

INTRODUCTION

Decreased bone mineral density is a spectrum of disease that must be considered by spine surgeons, as it has important implications on surgical interventions and patient outcomes. Osteoporosis presents as a quantitative decrease in bone mineralization. It is formally diagnosed using a dual x-ray absorptiometry (DEXA) bone scan or with a patient history of prior fragility fractures.[1] Osteoporosis most commonly affects postmenopausal women but is not limited to this demographic. The pathophysiology of osteoporosis involves various factors including aging, menopause, progressive inactivity, and decreased dietary calcium, all leading to thinner bone.[2]

Chin and colleagues conducted a cross-sectional study to determine the prevalence of osteoporosis among patients undergoing spine surgery. In their sample, they reported that among patients over the age of 50, 15% of men had osteoporosis, along with a staggering 50% of women.[3] These statistics emphasize why spine surgeons must be comfortable in managing these

patients. They also speak to how osteoporosis predisposes patients to fracture, spinal deformity, and spinal stenosis.[4] Thus, along with considering the disease as a patient comorbidity, osteoporosis also directly leads to spinal column pathology.

The primary examples of this are osteoporotic compression fractures, which are the most common fragility fracture seen in patients with decreased bone mineral density. These fractures occur most commonly in patients aged 60 to 70 years with decreased bone density and have complex treatment algorithms. Two hundred million people worldwide are affected by osteoporosis, and in the United States, 1.5 million osteoporotic fractures occur each year. These fractures include 700 thousand vertebral fractures, making these fractures among the most common pathologies seen by spine surgeon.[2] Both nonoperative management and surgical management play a role in treatment of these fractures.

This article reviews the appropriate assessment and management of osteoporotic compression fractures. It also discusses the implications

---

[a] LSU-HSC Department of Orthopaedics, 2021 Perdido Street, 7th Floor, New Orleans, LA 70112, USA; [b] LSU-HSC Department of Neurosurgery, 2021 Perdido Street, 7th Floor, New Orleans, LA 70112, USA
* Corresponding author.
E-mail address: dgelve@lsuhsc.edu

Orthop Clin N Am 55 (2024) 403–413
https://doi.org/10.1016/j.ocl.2024.01.001
0030-5898/24/© 2024 Elsevier Inc. All rights reserved.

of osteoporosis on initial patient evaluation, medical optimization for surgery, selection of instrumentation, and surgical technique. It further discusses adverse outcomes associated with osteoporosis. Failure to appropriately evaluate, optimize, and treat spine patients with osteoporotic bone can lead to disastrous complications. Weakened bone can lead to implant failure through cage subsidence and screw pullout. It can also lead to peri-implant fractures, failure of deformity correction, and proximal kyphosis. These risks must be taken into account when considering operative interventions in these patients, and surgical plans must be adapted accordingly. New advancements in spinal surgery allow surgeons to appropriately treat this population operatively with improved outcomes compared to patients with spinal pathology being managed nonoperatively.[4]

PATIENT EVALUATION

Recommendations for screening proposed by the World Health Organization (WHO) are for perimenopausal/postmenopausal women, those with known metabolic bone disease, and those with various known osteoporotic risk factors. These patients should be evaluated with a DEXA scan and metabolic laboratory testing. DEXA scan T scores of less than or equal to −2.5 are diagnostic of osteoporosis. Laboratory evaluation should include vitamin D3, calcium, serum alkaline phosphatase, osteocalcin, and measurement of collagen cross-link degradation in urine, which quantifies bone turnover.[5] Other less frequent laboratory tests are parathyroid hormone (PTH) and TSH, as these play a significant role in bone regulation and may be other causes of bone mineral disease (BMD). The National Osteoporosis Foundation (NOF) recommends screening with DEXA scan in women aged 65 and older and men aged 70 and older, postmenopausal women, men aged 50 to 69 with a risk factor profile, and all patients with known fragility fractures. A vertebral compression factor regardless of BMD is a diagnosis of osteoporosis and indicates need for treatment; given they may go undiagnosed for years, proactive vertebral imaging may be warranted. The NOF proposes vertebral imaging for

> Women older than 70 years and men aged 80 years and older
> Women aged 65 to 69 years and men aged 75 to 79 years if BMD is less than or equal to −1.5 (osteopenia)

> Postmenopausal women and men aged 50 to 69 years who have sustained a low energy fracture, previous height loss of greater than or equal to 4 cm, prospective height loss greater than or equal to 0.8 cm, or recent/long-term treatment with glucocorticoids.[6]

Prevention is the key principle in the treatment of osteoporosis and related fractures. Identifying at-risk populations allows earlier screening and initiation of therapies to prevent osteoporotic fractures. A detailed history and physical examination help to identify the at-risk population by assessing lifestyle factors, medical conditions, and physical patient characteristics that contribute to bone health and fracture risk. Identifiable risk factors that may contribute to bone health are caloric intake, appropriate dietary vitamin D and calcium intake, and physical exercise, as well as smoking status and amount of alcohol consumption.[5] The Fracture Risk Assessment tool (FRAX) was published by the WHO from the work and validation under the direction of Professor John Kanis; it was developed to calculate the probability of a low energy hip fracture and all other fragility fractures.[7,8]

Most patients undergoing spine surgery or being worked up for spine-related issues undergo a computed tomography (CT) scan or MRI. Recent evidence has suggested the use of Hounsfield units (HU) on CT to correlate with BMD and that they be used as a screening tool for osteoporosis.[9] Study by Au and colleagues described a significant correlation with T-scores less than or equal to −2.5 and HU means of 78.5 with standard deviation of 32.4.[10] MRI has not been shown to have significant effect in screening but does have a role in diagnosing occult fragility fractures, with a sensitivity of 75%, but is not very specific and lacks the ability to differentiate from neoplastic conditions.[11,12] MRI findings suggestive of fragility fractures are fracture lines, best seen on T1-weighted spin-echo sequences and bone marrow edema and on short tau inversion recovery sequences. For chronic fractures, there is usually more sclerosis, which is best appreciated on T1-weighted and short tau inversion sequences.[13]

PHARMACOLOGIC/MEDICAL TREATMENT OPTIONS AND MEDICAL OPTIMIZATION

Prevention and management of osteoporosis are key elements in reducing risk of osteoporotic vertebral fractures and in perioperative medical optimization. Poor bone quality can increase the risk of fixation failure with spinal instrumentation and cause delayed bone fusion.[14] Both antiresorptive and anabolic therapies play a role in the prevention of new osteoporotic fractures and in obtaining a good fusion rate in osteoporotic patients. Antiresorptive agents primarily inhibit osteoclast activity and bone resorption, while anabolic therapies primarily stimulate osteoblasts and bone formation. Patient education and regular control visits should be planned in a multidisciplinary manner to optimize medical management, maintain adherence to medication regimen, and mitigate potential risks to bony healing such as smoking.

Antiresorptive Treatments

Antiresorptive treatment modalities include calcium, vitamin D, selective estrogen receptor modulators (SERM), bisphosphonates, and receptor activator of NF-kB ligand (RANKL) antibody. The common characteristic of these drugs is inhibition of bone resorption, but the underlying mechanisms and pharmacodynamics of the drugs are variable.

Calcium and vitamin D have been the focus of many clinical studies investigating fracture prevention therapies. Antiresorptive mechanisms of action occur through stimulation of bone mineralization and suppression of serum levels of PTH. Modest antifracture efficacy has been demonstrated in meta-analyses of randomized control trials (RCTs).[15] A retrospective review conducted by Xu and colleagues suggests vitamin D3 supplementation alone may be sufficient to increase fusion rates in patients undergoing transforaminal lumbar interbody fusion (TLIF).[16] Calcium and vitamin D are considered central components of basic perioperative osteoporosis treatment and fracture prevention, and screening for vitamin D deficiency should be performed regularly for patients with undergoing spinal reconstructive surgery.

The prevalence of osteoporosis and related fractures is higher in postmenopausal women than in older men. SERMs were developed as an alternative to estrogen replacement therapy for prevention and treatment of postmenopausal osteoporosis.[17] The underlying mechanism involves binding to estrogen receptors in a different way than endogenous estrogen, thereby conferring protection against bone loss and osteoporosis without the adverse effect profile of estrogen replacement. SERMs continue to be investigated in large clinical trials with reported antifracture efficacy.[18] An animal model by Park and colleagues shows improved trabecular quality of the vertebral body, enhanced spinal fusion, and increased compact bone mass within the fusion bed, suggesting that SERMs may be useful to improve fusion rates in osteoporotic patients who undergo spinal surgery.[19]

Bisphosphonates are common anti-resorptive agents that promote apoptosis of mature osteoclasts and decrease the rate of bone remodeling.[20,21] Route of administration and affinity for bone are considered when selecting an appropriate treatment among several different agents. In animals, data regarding the effect of bisphosphonates on fusion rates are mixed; several studies show no adverse effects of bisphosphonates on fracture healing and pullout strength of implants,[22,23] while others demonstrate delayed spinal fusion.[24] Conversely, a human trial conducted by Nagahama and colleagues found significantly higher fusion rates in osteopenic patients undergoing single-level posterior lumbar interbody fusion with administration of alendronate postoperatively.[25] Furthermore, a meta-analysis by Liu and colleagues revealed that bisphosphonates improve lumbar fusion rate,[26] and a large cohort study by Guppy and colleagues found no effect of preoperative bisphosphonate use on operative nonunion rates in osteoporotic patients.[27] More recent meta-analyses have demonstrated benefits of bisphosphonate therapy in accelerating fusion postoperatively.[28,29] Although additional investigation is warranted to the determine the effect of preoperative and postoperative bisphosphonate on spinal fusion rates, clinical studies interpreted collectively do not support the cessation of bisphosphonate use perioperatively.

Denosumab is a monoclonal antibody to the receptor activator of NFKB ligand that blocks its binding to RANK. It inhibits the development and activity of osteoclasts, decreasing bone resorption, and increasing bone density.[18,21,30] RCTs have shown denosumab to demonstrate efficacy against vertebral and nonvertebral fractures in women with osteoporosis[18] and improve bony union and spinal fusion rates in combination with teriparatide.[30] Other anti-resorptive agents such as cathepsin K inhibitors and integrin $\alpha\nu\beta3$ antagonists have been found to increase bone mass and inhibit osteoclastic resorption.[21] Although these novel treatments hold promise in the treatment of osteoporosis, further investigation into the effects of antiresorptive therapies on spine fusion are required.

Anabolic Treatments

Anabolic treatments of osteoporosis are comprised of PTH analogs. Studies have shown that short-term elevation in serum PTH result in increased osteoblastic activity, whereas long-term elevation in serum PTH results in increased osteoblastic and osteoclastic activity that ultimately leads to increased bone turnover.

Teriparatide (Forteo) is a PTH-related peptide analog that binds to the teriparatide receptor, preferentially activating and stimulating osteoblasts over osteoclasts.[20] Teriparatide is given as a daily subcutaneous injection to rapidly stimulate bone formation; it has been shown to mitigate vertebral and nonvertebral fracture risk in postmenopausal women with osteoporosis and glucocorticoid-induced osteoporosis.[31,32] Animal studies on intermittent PTH treatment suggest improvement in fusion rate and fusion mass microstructure.[20] An RCT by Ebata and colleagues demonstrated enhanced interbody fusion rates in elderly women treated with TLIF/PLIF.[33] Investigations have consistently demonstrated shorter mean interbody fusion duration with teriparatide treatment and significantly reduced number of screw loosening events.[30,34,35] Several recent meta-analyses have corroborated the effectiveness of teriparatide therapy, resulting in higher fusion rates following lumbar spinal surgery.[28,29,36]

Abaloparatide (Tymlos) is a new peptide that also binds to the teriparatide receptor with similar downstream effects. Differences in this binding have been shown to result in less osteoclast activation than teriparatide.[33] A large clinical trial demonstrated that although both drugs mitigate fracture risk, abaloparatide showed a stronger increase in BMD in the hip region and the lumbar spine.[37] The clinical implications of this increase in BMD with regard to spinal fusion have yet to be determined.

Smoking Cessation

Smoking has been identified as a risk factor for osteoporosis, fractures, and increased complications following spinal fusion. Tobacco smoke influences bone mass directly through effects on osteogenesis and angiogenesis of bone. Recent evidence demonstrates that tobacco smoking causes an imbalance in bone turnover, leading to lower bone mass and increasing risk of osteoporotic fractures.[38] It has been demonstrated that smoking increases the rate of perioperative complications for patients undergoing spinal fusion surgery, with a twofold greater rate of pseudarthrosis following lumbar or cervical surgery.[39] Investigations are ongoing as to whether nicotine replacement therapy may be a preferred alternative to smoking. The current recommendation is cessation of smoking at least 4 to 6 weeks before spinal fusion surgery.

Multidisciplinary Approach to Medical Management

Treatment methods for osteoporotic patients requiring spinal fusion is a growing field of interest. Multimodal solutions are now available that involve the employment of osteoporosis medications to increase BMD and modification of lifestyle choices that induce bone resorption. Best practice guidelines have been developed by an expert multidisciplinary panel to identify and treat patients with poor bone health before elective spinal reconstruction.[40] All patients above 65 and those under 65 with particular risk factors should have formal bone health evaluation before undergoing surgery. The literature most strongly supports anabolic agents as first-line therapy to decrease postoperative complications and increase fusion rate.[28–30,34–36] However, anti-resorptive agents are acceptable alternatives in the event of a contraindication to anabolic agents. Medical management should be initiated preoperatively for at least 2 months and postoperatively for a minimum of 8 months.[40] Consultation with a bone health physician and relevant subspecialty medical services should be considered on an individual basis to collaborate in managing osteoporosis. Increasing awareness and treatment of osteoporosis can improve outcomes and prevent complications for patients undergoing spinal fusion surgery.

SURGICAL CONSIDERATIONS

In the population aged greater than 50, the reported incidence of osteopenia was 46.1% and 41.4% for men and women.[3] With advanced age, comorbidities that increase overall surgical risk often exist. In the osteoporotic spine, bone-implant failure is most commonly the result of screw cutout/pullout, and optimizing this interface is paramount.[2] It is important to maximize strength of fixation to compensate for weaker bone. Decreased BMD has been shown to correlate with failure of thoracolumbar instrumentation.[41] This means optimizing fixation technique and using increasing points of fixation. Increasing points of fixation is thought to dissipate the forces throughout the spine.[4] Hybrid constructs that use sublaminar wires and laminar hooks in addition to traditional pedicle screws may increase pullout strength and improve overall stability.[42,43] Various surgical techniques can improve fixation and facilitate union in the osteoporotic spine; this includes consideration of the construct length, fusion and pedicle screw technique, and cement augmentation.[44–56]

Posterior Instrumentation

Traditional pedicle screw positioning and insertion techniques have been extensively studied to optimize pullout strength. For example, Lehman and colleagues reported that in the thoracic spine, maximal insertional torque and pullout strength may be increased by placing screws in a straight-forward direction rather than anatomic trajectory.[57] Pedicle screw insertion angled toward subchondral bone also follows for stronger fixation and insertional torque.[58] Oversizing screws should be avoided, as larger screws against the thinned pedicle cortices encountered in osteoporosis may predispose to fracture. Helgeson and colleagues reported the inferior portion of pedicle provides the most robust fixation, and under-tapping increases pullout strength. The sizing and positioning of these screws are crucial for attaining optimal fixation.[59] Placement depth of these screws also has biomechanical implications, with many surgeons preferring to hub pedicle screws against the dorsolaminar cortex. Paik and colleagues demonstrated this resulted in significantly lower pullout strength in osteoporotic vertebrae.[60] They also similarly reported the use of rod reduction devices decreased pullout strength and encouraged further rod contouring or adjustment of pedicle screw depth.[61] Additional strategies including hydroxyapatite coating of pedicle screws are currently being studied in animal models.[62]

Cement Augmentation and Fenestrated Screws

Cement augmentation of pedicle screws has been extensively studied and can stand to increase pullout strength by up to 149%.[44,63] Chen and colleagues reported cement augmentation decreased loss of deformity correction and higher fusion rate.[64] Sawakami and colleagues reported similar results in terms of decreased radiographic lucency, correction loss, and fusion rate. Solid screws with retrograde cement filling appear to have higher pullout strength than cannulated or fenestrated screws; however, this technique has also been reported to require longer operative times with higher rates of cement leakage.[63,64]

Prophylactic vertebroplasty may reduce the rate of junctional failure by reducing the stiffness between end of construct and adjacent level.[65] Patients with caudal and cephalad vertebroplasty have lower rates of screw loosening, mechanical failure, and junctional segment fractures.[66]

Level Selection

Level selection becomes only more critical in the management of the osteoporotic spine. Affected levels should be identified and sagittal alignment restored. However, aggressive correction in patients older than 60 increases the risk of junctional kyphosis.[58,67]

Longer constructs provide increased points of fixation and avoid junctional or segmental failure, with Dodwad and colleagues recommending at least 3 levels proximal and distal to distribute strain across multiple points of fixation.[58]

In osteoporotic bone, proximal junctional strain is increased. Junctional strain at the upper instrumented level of the construct may lead to accelerated and progressive deformity. Transitional junctions including the cervicothoracic and thoracolumbar junction should be avoided because of their predisposition for kyphotic collapse. For example, instrumenting the L1 level should be avoided, and these constructs should be taken to T10.[67]

Prior studies have described always instrumenting 3 levels above and below the apex of the deformity and never instrumenting at a kyphotic level.[58]

With regards to the lower instrumented level, use of iliac and/or sacral fixation is recommended whenever possible. This reduces sacral insufficiency fractures, increases construct stability, reduces pseudarthrosis, and reduces implant failure. S2 alar-iliac screws have lower implant prominence and lower complication rate than traditional iliac fixation.[42] Some authors have suggested that instrumenting the pelvis with 4 screws as opposed to 2 can further increase fixation strength in osteoporotic bone.[68]

Interbody Versus No Interbody

Interbody instrumentation and fusion allow for indirect decompression of the spinal canal and neuroforaminal space. Less invasive techniques involving interbody instrumentation including minimally invasive surgery (MIS) TLIF, OLIF, ALIF, LLIF, and PTP interbody fusion have continued to gain traction as important techniques for treating spinal and neuroforaminal stenosis without the morbidity of open decompression.[69] However, these procedures carry their own complications, including incomplete relief of stenosis, cage subsidence, and the morbidity of the different lateral or anterior approaches. Therefore, careful patient selection for these techniques is pivotal. Yingsakmongkol and colleagues conducted a retrospective review in 191 patients who underwent LLIF and identified 4 important criteria for determining if patients would benefit from indirect decompression:

1. Dynamic clinical symptoms with pain relief in the supine position
2. Reducible disc height with improved disc height in the supine position
3. Absence of profound weakness
4. Absence of static stenosis

In patients who met these criteria, more than 93% had successful outcomes with indirect decompression. When applying these considerations to the osteoporotic patient, several factors come into play (Fig. 1). Patients with osteoporosis tend to be older with more degenerated spines due not only to their age, but also weakened bone.[4] This pathology can lead to more severe stenosis and neurologic symptoms (points 3 and 4 of criteria for successful indirect decompression). More severe degeneration can also lead to locked, immobile facets that do not allow for positional correction of disc height.

Another important consideration when it comes to interbody fusion in the osteoporotic patient is cage subsidence. Cage subsidence occurs when the interbody instrumentation violates the end plate over time, leading to loss of correction from the indirect decompression procedure. In their study, Yingsakmongkol and colleagues identified low BMD (T-score < -2.1) as being associated with failure of indirect decompression. Morgan and colleagues reviewed 120 patients who underwent LLIF. There was a 4.1% failure rate of indirect decompression requiring secondary decompression. All of the patients underwent standalone LLIF, and most had evidence of osteoporosis. However, the group as a whole had 60% of patients with osteoporosis many of whom had some small level of interbody graft subsidence. Several studies have been done on fusion rates for interbody fusion in the osteoporotic patient. Patients older than 70 who underwent PLIF had a higher rate of delayed union but not a statistically significant rate of overall fusion. In combination, these data suggest that osteoporosis is a risk factor for failure of indirect decompression and graft subsidence. However, with supplemental pedicle screw instrumentation in addition to interbody fusion and careful endplate preparation, it can still be a successful technique in osteoporotic patients with favorable outcomes greater than 90% demonstrated in studies.[70] Furthermore, patient-reported outcomes in multiple areas improve substantially following surgery even in this population.[51] However, postponing elective spine procedures to allow for medical optimization remains controversial, as several studies have suggested that delays in surgical treatment way predispose to worse clinical outcomes.[52]

Minimally Invasive Surgery Versus Open

Interbody indirect decompression techniques are frequently combined with percutaneous pedicle screw placement to allow for a minimally invasive approach to decompression of the spine. In contrast, open approaches involve direct decompression by removing compressive posterior spinal column elements through larger incisions with more muscular dissection. Park and colleagues analyzed how spine surgeons decide on minimally invasive approaches versus open approaches in patients with spinal deformity. They looked at 268 patients, 120 of whom underwent open surgery and 148 whom underwent MIS. The authors found that the primary factor in surgeons opting for a minimally invasive approach was age.[71] This finding is interesting given patients with increased age are more likely to have osteoporosis and have more issues with indirect decompression. However, the risks of interbody fusion in osteoporotic bone must be balanced on the other comorbidities seen in older patients. Older patients tend to be more frail and have more medical comorbidities that may be less exacerbated by minimally invasive approaches.

Park and colleagues also found that spine surgeons tend to opt for open approaches in patients with more severe deformity and compression. Patients with osteoporosis will frequently tend to have more severe pathology because weaker bone leading to more significant deformity.[4] However, this is not necessarily a linear relationship. There are studies showing that patients with increased BMDs tend to have more significant osteophyte formation, disc degeneration, end plate sclerosis, and spondylolisthesis.[72] Thus, the relationship between osteoporosis and spinal deformity is complex, and treatment plans should be individualized to patients.

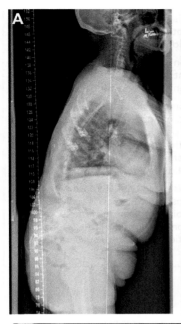
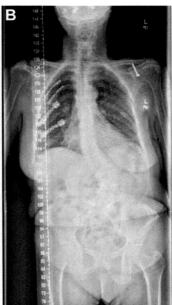

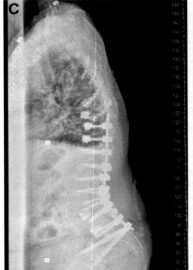
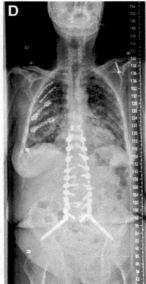

Fig. 1. (*A*) Lateral full-length spinal film of osteoporotic patient with significant spinal deformity with large positive sagittal balance. (*B*) Anterior-posterior (AP) full-length spinal film of same patient showing significant coronal deformity. (*C*) Postoperative lateral full-length film demonstrating use of multiple lumbar interbody fusions, pelvic instrumentation, fenestrated screws at the 2 highest instrumented levels with cement augmentation, and kyphoplasty at the level above. Appropriate sagittal balance restored. (*D*) Postoperative full-length AP film showing impressive coronal correction.

Frequently, surgeons will use interbody techniques during open procedures to improve spinal alignment, apply further decompression, and increase rate of fusion through anterior column instrumentation. When considering this technique in patients with decreased BMD, selection of the number and levels to which the interbody cages are applied is important. Two-thirds of the lordosis of the lumbar spine come from L4-L5, and L5-S1, making these levels the most important to target with interbody cages when performing large corrective surgeries. While adding additional interbody spacers can help improve spinal alignment, fusion rates, and decompression of the spine, it can lead to increased risk of complications in older patients with decreased BMD. More interbody cages in weak bone may lead to increased risk of end plate violation and subsidence. Performing interbody fusion at more levels will also increase operative time, which increases overall risk of surgery, especially in older more frail patients.[66]

DISCUSSION/FUTURE DIRECTION/ SUMMARY

As the general population continues to age, osteoporosis will continue to be a large factor in surgical planning for spine surgery. Weakened bone in patients with osteoporosis leads directly to spinal deformity. Therefore, these patients make up a significant portion of the population encountered by spine surgeons. It is important to work closely with endocrinologists and primary care physicians to optimize these patients for any surgical intervention. These patients are at higher risk for complications during surgery including fracture, interbody cage subsidence, and implant failure.

However, many studies have shown that patients with osteoporosis can still have favorable outcomes with spine surgery. Strategies for optimizing these outcomes include fenestrated screws with cement augmentation, increasing points of fixation with more aggressive level selection, screw placement technique, less aggressive coronal plane deformity correction, and implementation of minimally invasive techniques in appropriate patients.

Technological advancements including fenestrated screws, expandable screws, navigation, and pedicle screws with coating specific for osteoporotic bone are furthering spine surgeons' ability to adequately treat this more delicate population. Continuing advancements in PMMA cement and newer types of cement are being implemented for increased fixation. There is cement and screw coating being developed with biologic properties for optimizing bony ingrowth. Newer screw techniques including bicortical screws, crossing screws, undertapping screws, and double screw techniques have been shown to have biomechanical advantages in osteoporotic bone. Lastly, there are new implants being developed with tantalum, which has a higher modulus of elasticity and excellent bony ingrowth and biocompatibility.

Although novel, most of these techniques have promising biomechanical data. As strategies, techniques, and implants continue to advance in the field of spine surgery, surgeons will need to continue their education in order to optimally treat osteoporotic patients with spinal pathology.[73]

CLINICS CARE POINTS

- Osteoporosis leads to spinal deformity, stenosis, and fractures.

- Osteoporosis is diagnosed with a dual x-ray absorptiometry scan in at-risk patients, especially older women.

- Patients can be optimized with medical management with bisphosphonates, vitamin D supplementation, and teriparatide.

- Vertebral compression fractures can primarily be managed nonoperatively. If there is progressive pain, deformity, or neurologic symptoms, they can be managed with vertebroplasty, kyphoplasty, or posterior instrumentation/fusion.

- Osteoporosis carries increased risk of complications, but techniques such as increased points of fixation, cement augmentation, and optimizing posterior instrumentation can lead to successful outcomes.

DISCLOSURE

The authors of this review article have no pertinent disclosures or conflicts of interest.

REFERENCES

1. Jeremiah MP, Unwin BK, Greenawald MH, et al. Diagnosis and management of osteoporosis. Am Fam Physician 2015;92(4):261–8.
2. Matzkin EG, DeMaio M, Charles JF, et al. Diagnosis and treatment of osteoporosis: what orthopaedic surgeons need to know. J Am Acad Orthop Surg 2019;27(20):E902–12.
3. Chin DK, Park JY, Yoon YS, et al. Prevalence of osteoporosis in patients requiring spine surgery: incidence and significance of osteoporosis in spine disease. Osteoporos Int 2007;18(9):1219–24.
4. Tomé-Bermejo F, Piñera AR, Alvarez L. Osteoporosis and the management of spinal degenerative disease (II). Arch Bone Jt Surg 2017;5(6):363–74.
5. Lane JM, Nydick M. Osteoporosis: current modes of prevention and treatment. J Am Acad Orthop Surg 1999;7(1):19–31.
6. Cosman F, de Beur SJ, LeBoff MS, et al. Clinician's guide to prevention and treatment of osteoporosis. Osteoporos Int 2014;25(10):2359–81.
7. Kanis JA, Johnell O, Oden A, et al. FRAX™ and the assessment of fracture probability in men and women from the UK. Osteoporos Int 2008;19(4):385–97.
8. Kanis JA. Assessment of osteoporosis at the primary health care level. World Health. 2007:339. Available at: http://www.shef.ac.uk/FRAX/pdfs/WHO_Technical_Report.pdf.
9. Kim KJ, Kim DH, Lee J II, et al. Hounsfield units on lumbar computed tomography for predicting

regional bone mineral density. Open Med 2019;14: 545–51.

10. Schreiber JJ, Anderson PA, Rosas HG, et al. Hounsfield units for assessing bone mineral density and strength: a tool for osteoporosis management. J Bone Jt Surg 2011;93(11):1057–63.

11. Cabarrus MC, Ambekar A, Lu Y, et al. MRI and CT of insufficiency fractures of the pelvis and the proximal femur. Am J Roentgenol 2008;191(4):995–1001.

12. Graham-Gotis L, McGuigan L, Diamond T, et al. Sacral insufficiency fractures in the elderly. J Bone Jt Surg - Ser B 1994;76(6):882–6.

13. Link TM. Radiology of osteoporosis. Can Assoc Radiol J 2016;67(1):28–40.

14. DeWald CJ, Stanley T. Instrumentation-related complications of multilevel fusions for adult spinal deformity patients over age 65: surgical considerations and treatment options in patients with poor bone quality. Spine (Phila Pa 1976) 2006; 31(19 Suppl):144–51.

15. Bischoff-Ferrari HA, Willett WC, Wong JB, et al. Prevention of nonvertebral fractures with oral vitamin D and dose dependency: a meta-analysis of randomized controlled trials. Arch Intern Med 2009;169(6):551–61.

16. Xu Y, Zhou M, Liu H, et al. Effect of 1,25-dihydroxyvitamin D3 on posterior transforaminal lumbar interbody fusion in patients with osteoporosis and lumbar disc degenerative disease. Zhongguo Xiu Fu Chong Jian Wai Ke Za Zhi 2014;28(8): 969–72.

17. Silverman SL, Christiansen C, Genant HK, et al. Efficacy of bazedoxifene in reducing new vertebral fracture risk in postmenopausal women with osteoporosis: results from a 3-year, randomized, placebo-, and active-controlled clinical trial. J Bone Miner Res 2008;23(12):1923–34.

18. Cummings SR, Martin JS, McClung MR, et al. Denosumab for prevention of fractures in postmenopausal women with osteoporosis. Obstet Gynecol Surv 2009;64(12):805–7.

19. Park SB, Kim CH, Hong M, et al. Effect of a selective estrogen receptor modulator on bone formation in osteoporotic spine fusion using an ovariectomized rat model. Spine J 2016;16(1):72–81.

20. Hirsch BP, Unnanuntana A, Cunningham ME, et al. The effect of therapies for osteoporosis on spine fusion: a systematic review. Spine J 2013;13(2): 190–9.

21. Roux S. New treatment targets in osteoporosis. Jt Bone Spine 2010;77(3):222–8.

22. Nakamura Y, Hayashi K, Abu-Ali S, et al. Effect of preoperative combined treatment with alendronate and calcitriol on fixation of hydroxyapatite-coated implants in ovariectomized rats. J Bone Jt Surg 2008;90(4):824–32.

23. Takahata M, Ito M, Abe Y, et al. The effect of anti-resorptive therapies on bone graft healing in an ovariectomized rat spinal arthrodesis model. Bone 2008;43(6):1057–66.

24. Huang RC, Khan SN, Sandhu HS, et al. Alendronate inhibits spine fusion in a rat model. Spine (Phila Pa 1976) 2005;30(22):2516–22.

25. Nagahama K, Kanayama M, Togawa D, et al. Does alendronate disturb the healing process of posterior lumbar interbody fusion? A prospective randomized trial. J Neurosurg Spine 2011;14(4):500–7.

26. Liu W Bin, Zhao WT, Shen P, et al. The effects of bisphosphonates on osteoporotic patients after lumbar fusion: a meta-analysis. Drug Des Devel Ther 2018;12:2233–40.

27. Guppy KH, Chan PH, Prentice HA, et al. Does the use of preoperative bisphosphonates in patients with osteopenia and osteoporosis affect lumbar fusion rates? Analysis from a national spine registry. Neurosurg Focus 2020;49(2):1–10.

28. Tsai SHL, Chien R-S, Lichter K, et al. Teriparatide and bisphosphonate use in osteoporotic spinal fusion patients: a systematic review and meta-analysis. Arch Osteoporosis 2020;15(1):158.

29. Govindarajan V, Diaz A, Perez-Roman RJ, et al. Osteoporosis treatment in patients undergoing spinal fusion: a systematic review and meta-analysis. Neurosurg Focus 2021;50(6):1–11.

30. Ide M, Yamada K, Kaneko K, et al. Combined teriparatide and denosumab therapy accelerates spinal fusion following posterior lumbar interbody fusion. Orthop Traumatol Surg Res 2018;104(7): 1043–8.

31. Neer RM, Arnaud CD, Zanchetta JR, et al. Effect of parathyroid hormone (1-34) on fractures and bone mineral density in postmenopausal women with osteoporosis. N Engl J Med 2001;344(19):1434–41.

32. Aspenberg P, Malouf J, Tarantino U, et al. Effects of teriparatide compared with risedronate on recovery after pertrochanteric hip fracture results of a randomized, active-controlled, double-blind clinical trial at 26 weeks. J Bone Jt Surg - Am 2016; 98(22):1868–78.

33. Boyce EG, Mai Y, Pham C. Abaloparatide: review of a next-generation parathyroid hormone agonist. Ann Pharmacother 2018;52(5):462–72.

34. Yolcu YU, Zreik J, Alvi MA, et al. Use of teriparatide prior to lumbar fusion surgery lowers two-year complications for patients with poor bone health. Clin Neurol Neurosurg 2020;198(September): 106244.

35. Kim JW, Park SW, Kim YB, et al. The effect of postoperative use of teriparatide reducing screw loosening in osteoporotic patients. J Korean Neurosurg Soc 2018;61(4):494–502.

36. Fatima N, Massaad E, Hadzipasic M, et al. Assessment of the efficacy of teriparatide treatment for

osteoporosis on lumbar fusion surgery outcomes: a systematic review and meta-analysis. Neurosurg Rev 2021;44(3):1357–70.

37. Leder BZ, O'Dea LSL, Zanchetta JR, et al. Effects of abaloparatide, a human parathyroid hormone-related peptide analog, on bone mineral density in postmenopausal women with osteoporosis. J Clin Endocrinol Metab 2015;100(2):697–706.

38. Al-Bashaireh AM, Haddad LG, Weaver M, et al. The effect of tobacco smoking on bone mass: an overview of pathophysiologic mechanisms. J Osteoporos 2018;2018.

39. Khurana VG. Adverse impact of smoking on the spine and spinal surgery. Surg Neurol Int 2021;12:118.

40. Sardar ZM, Coury JR, Cerpa M, et al. Best practice guidelines for assessment and management of osteoporosis in adult patients undergoing elective spinal reconstruction. Spine (Phila Pa 1976) 2022;47(2):128–35.

41. Lau D, Clark AJ, Scheer JK, et al. Proximal junctional kyphosis and failure after spinal deformity surgery: a systematic review of the literature as a background to classification development. Spine (Phila Pa 1976) 2014;39(25):2093–102.

42. Kebaish KM. Sacropelvic fixation: techniques and complications. Spine (Phila Pa 1976) 2010;35(25):2245–51.

43. Kanno H, Onoda Y, Hashimoto, et al. Innovation of surgical techniques for screw fixation in patients with osteoporotic spine. J Clin Med 2022;11(9).

44. Lehman RA, Kang DG, Wagner SC. Management of osteoporosis in spine surgery. J Am Acad Orthop Surg 2015;23(4):253–63.

45. Knopp-Sihota JA, Newburn-Cook CV, Homik J, et al. Calcitonin for treating acute and chronic pain of recent and remote osteoporotic vertebral compression fractures: a systematic review and meta-analysis. Osteoporos Int 2012;23(1):17–38.

46. Esses SI, McGuire R, Jenkins J, et al. The treatment of symptomatic osteoporotic spinal compression fractures. J Am Acad Orthop Surg 2011;19(3):176–82.

47. Imamudeen N, Basheer A, Iqbal AM, et al. Management of osteoporosis and spinal fractures: contemporary guidelines and evolving paradigms. Clin Med Res 2022;20(2):95–106.

48. Beall D, Lorio MP, Min Yun B, et al. Review of vertebral augmentation: an updated metaanalysis of the effectiveness. Internet J Spine Surg 2018;12(3):295–321.

49. Hirsch JA, Chandra RV, Carter NS, et al. Number needed to treat with vertebral augmentation to save a life. Am J Neuroradiol 2020;41(1):178–82.

50. Barr JD, Jensen ME, Hirsch JA, et al. Position statement on percutaneous vertebral augmentation: a consensus statement developed by the society of interventional radiology (SIR), American Association of Neurological Surgeons (AANS) and the Congress of Neurological Surgeons (CNS), American College of Radiology (ACR). J Vasc Intervent Radiol 2014;25(2):171–81.

51. Anderson PA, Froyshteter AB, Tontz WL. Meta-analysis of vertebral augmentation compared with conservative treatment for osteoporotic spinal fractures. J Bone Miner Res 2013;28(2):372–82.

52. McGraw JK, Lippert JA, Minkus KD, et al. Prospective evaluation of pain relief in 100 patients undergoing percutaneous vertebroplasty: results and follow-up. J Vasc Intervent Radiol 2002;13(9 I):883–6.

53. Diamond TH, Champion B, Clark WA. Management of acute osteoporotic vertebral fractures: a nonrandomized trial comparing percutaneous vertebroplasty with conservative therapy. Am J Med 2003;114(4):257–65.

54. Xu Z, Hao D, Dong L, et al. Surgical options for symptomatic old osteoporotic vertebral compression fractures: a retrospective study of 238 cases. BMC Surg 2021;21(1):1–10.

55. Alpantaki K, Dohm M, Korovessis P, et al. Surgical options for osteoporotic vertebral compression fractures complicated with spinal deformity and neurologic deficit. Injury 2018;49(2):261–71.

56. Kim SK, Chung JY, Park YJ, et al. Modified pedicle subtraction osteotomy for osteoporotic vertebral compression fractures. Orthop Surg 2020;388–95.

57. Lehman RA, Polly DW, Kuklo TR, et al. Straight-forward versus anatomic trajectory technique of thoracic pedicle screw fixation: a biomechanical analysis. Spine (Phila Pa 1976) 2003;28(18):2058–65.

58. Dodwad SNM, Khan SN. Surgical stabilization of the spine in the osteoporotic patient. Orthop Clin N Am 2013;44(2):243–9.

59. Helgeson MD, Kang DG, Lehman RA, et al. Tapping insertional torque allows prediction for better pedicle screw fixation and optimal screw size selection. Spine J 2013;13(8):957–65.

60. Paik H, Dmitriev AE, Lehman RA, et al. The biomechanical effect of pedicle screw hubbing on pullout resistance in the thoracic spine. Spine J 2012;12(5):417–24.

61. Paik H, Kang DG, Lehman RA, et al. The biomechanical consequences of rod reduction on pedicle screws: should it be avoided? Spine J 2013;13(11):1617–26.

62. Hasegawa T, Inufusa A, Imai Y, et al. Hydroxyapatite-coating of pedicle screws improves resistance against pull-out force in the osteoporotic canine lumbar spine model: a pilot study. Spine J 2005;5(3):239–43.

63. Chang MC, Kao HC, Ying SH, et al. Polymethylmethacrylate augmentation of cannulated pedicle screws for fixation in osteoporotic spines and

comparison of its clinical results and biomechanical characteristics with the needle injection method. J Spinal Disord Tech 2013;26(6):305–15.

64. Chen LH, Tai CL, Lee DM, et al. Pullout strength of pedicle screws with cement augmentation in severe osteoporosis: a comparative study between cannulated screws with cement injection and solid screws with cement pre-filling. BMC Muscoskel Disord 2011;12:1–11.

65. Wenger M, Markwalder TM. Vertebroplasty combined with pedicular instrumentation. J Clin Neurosci 2008;15(3):257–62.

66. Ponnusamy KE, Iyer S, Gupta G, et al. Instrumentation of the osteoporotic spine: Biomechanical and clinical considerations. Spine J 2011;11(1): 54–63.

67. Kim HJ, Bridwell KH, Lenke LG, et al. Patients with proximal junctional kyphosis requiring revision surgery have higher postoperative lumbar lordosis and larger sagittal balance corrections. Spine (Phila Pa 1976) 2014;39(9):576–80.

68. Shen FH, Mason JR, Shimer AL, et al. Pelvic fixation for adult scoliosis. Eur Spine J 2013;22(Suppl 2): S265–75.

69. McKeithan LJ, Romano JW, Waddell WH, et al. Outcomes following direct versus indirect decompression techniques for lumbar spondylolisthesis: a propensity-matched analysis. Spine (Phila Pa 1976) 2022;47(20):1443–51.

70. Morgan CD, Walker CT, Godzik J, et al. When indirect decompression fails: a review of 220 consecutive direct lateral interbody fusions and unplanned secondary decompression. Spine (Phila Pa 1976) 2021;46(16):1081–6.

71. Park P, Than KD, Mummaneni PV, et al. Factors affecting approach selection for minimally invasive versus open surgery in the treatment of adult spinal deformity: analysis of a prospective, nonrandomized multicenter study. J Neurosurg Spine 2020; 33(5):601–6.

72. Paiva LC, Filardi S, Pinto-Neto AM, et al. Impact of degenerative radiographic abnormalities and vertebral fractures on spinal bone density of women with osteoporosis. Sao Paulo Med J 2002; 120(1):9–12.

73. Tandon V, Franke J, Kalidindi KKV. Advancements in osteoporotic spine fixation. J Clin Orthop Trauma 2020;11(5):778–85.

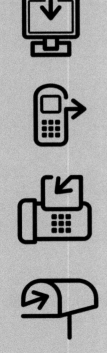